Sports Nutrition Strategies for Success

Sports Nutrition Strategies for Success

A Practical Guide to Improving Performance Through Nutrition

Abigail J. Larson
Kary Woodruff

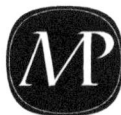

MP MOMENTUM PRESS
HEALTH

Sports Nutrition Strategies for Success: A Practical Guide to Improving Performance Through Nutrition
Copyright © Momentum Press®, LLC, 2017

First published in 2017 by
Momentum Press®, LLC
222 East 46th Street, New York, NY 10017
www.momentumpress.net

ISBN-13: 978-1-94474-997-2 (print)
ISBN-13: 978-1-94474-998-9 (e-book)

Momentum Press Health, Wellness, and Exercise Science Collection

Cover and interior design by S4Carlisle Publishing Services Private Ltd., Chennai, India

First edition: 2017
10 9 8 7 6 5 4 3 2 1

Printed in the United States of America

Dedication

To DK—thanks for everything and to Henry who forfeited a lot of playground and pool time this year.

KW—To Eric who always encourages and supports my passions. I couldn't do this without you. Evelyn and Nora you two support your mother in ways you cannot understand!

Abstract

The intent of this book is to provide science-based nutrition recommendations that will support optimal performance as well as promote the health and well-being of the athlete. The reader can expect an overview of sports nutrition fundamentals, including a breakdown of the macronutrient (carbohydrates, proteins, and fats), micronutrient, and hydration recommendations. Optimal quantity and timing of nutrient intake is also addressed. This information is then expanded upon through applied scenarios and strategies intended to help the reader develop individualized sports nutrition and hydration *plans* which implement recommendations within the context of busy schedules. This text also addresses weight management issues and how to best support athletes in achieving healthy weight gain or weight loss goals; disordered eating and eating disorders prevention, risks, signs, symptoms, and treatments among athletes; and risks and benefits of dietary supplements (including a helpful risk and application schemata for common dietary supplements); finally this text concludes with a chapter devoted to delicious and nutritious meal and snack recipes and a list of reputable resources for further reading. Ultimately this text is intended to be a practical, meaningful, and applied sport nutrition resource for exercise professionals across a wide range of disciplines.

Keywords

Adolescent Athletes, Coaches Education, Dietary Needs, Exercise Performance, Exercise Science, Meal Planning, Sports Nutrition, Sport Performance

Contents

Preface

Athletic success is the result of a myriad of factors, only some of which are controllable. Genetics and luck are beyond the control of the athlete, but appropriate training, rest, and dietary practices allow an athlete the opportunity to reach his or her potential. Nutrition, though often overlooked, is especially important for the young developing athlete. Adolescence and young adulthood is a time of rapid physical development. Young bodies can adapt to the demands of training quickly, but these adaptations can only happen and persist under the right circumstances: optimal training progression, optimal rest, and optimal nutrition. If any of these pieces are missing an athlete can easily become stale, ill, injured, overtrained, or just plainly underperform. It is only through optimally *fueling* the body that one can optimally *train* the body. It is only through optimal training that one can reach their athletic potential.

Consider the athlete who is *not* practicing optimal nutrition strategies. This includes the athlete who arrives to morning practice or a game without having eaten breakfast, or the athlete who trains after school on an empty stomach. These athletes are visibly tired and lethargic. Speed and agility, focus and concentration are hindered. Or consider the athlete playing a 90-minute soccer game who neglects to refuel or hydrate during the game. In the second half of the game this player covers less area of the field, has poor strategic judgement, and diminished accuracy. There is also the example of the athlete trying to make weight for a wrestling match. This individual has restricted energy intake for days and has not consumed any fluids for over 24 hours. He makes his goal weight, but his performance in the match is abysmal and he is at risk for considerable medical complications. These examples show how poor nutrition and hydration habits significantly and negatively affect the physical and cognitive performance of the athlete.

Eating is an integral component of daily sport practices. Just as young athletes need help training, many also need guidance as to how to eat for performance. As such, it is important that coaches, physical educators, athletic trainers, and all those who help athletes, be able to answer basic nutrition queries as well as have an understanding of how to best feed their hungry athletes before, during, and after play. Also important for individuals working with athletes is the ability to identify nutrition-related problems and act appropriately.

Sports Nutrition Strategies for Success: A Practical Guide to Improving Performance through Nutrition is intended to introduce the reader to sports nutrition recommendations and practices. Specifically this text will outline optimal fueling practices for young athletes and practical means of application. The primary objective of this book is to distill how training affects nutrient demands, how to meet these demands, and how optimal, as well as less than optimal, fueling practices can affect short- and long-term sport performance and health. Presented information includes basic macro- and micronutrient functions and recommendations, appropriate timing of food and fluid intake, strategic and individualized meal and snack planning, evidence-based methods and strategies to decrease fat mass and/or increase lean body mass, eating disorders in athletes, risks and benefits of common supplements and ergogenic aids, and recipes to meet activity-based energy and nutrient requirements as well as additional resources for further reading on specific topics of interest.

Ultimately by learning and sharing the tools and concepts presented in this text, you can help athletes take personal interest in developing and maintaining healthy eating habits for a lifetime.

Acknowledgment

KW and AL—We would like to acknowledge the contributions and information contributed from Kristi Spence, MS, RD, CSSD. Kristi has been a part of this book in many ways and we appreciate all of her wisdom and support. And thanks to Michelle Openshaw, MS, RD who recognized the need and inspired the conception of this text.

CHAPTER 1

Basic Sports Nutrition Guidelines

Introduction

Having a solid understanding of credible sports nutrition information allows athletes to make educated choices about how to properly fuel their bodies to support optimal performance. Unfortunately, athletes often turn to the Internet and other media sources for sports nutrition information that is not based on the most recent scientific research. This chapter provides an overview of the three macronutrients that provide energy to athletes (carbohydrates, proteins, and fats) and a summary of how the body utilizes this energy. Next it describes the micronutrients (vitamins and minerals) that serve multiple functions in the body and their relevance to athletic performance. Finally, there is an explanation of the role of proper hydration and recommendations for effective hydration strategies. This chapter also addresses practical information regarding the timing of intake so that athletes have an understanding of how to apply this information to improve performance.

Energy from Macronutrients

Humans obtain energy in the form of food, specifically the dietary *macronutrients* carbohydrates, proteins, and fat. In turn, the release of this stored potential energy allows for basic biological processes as well as more advanced functions such as running and moving heavy objects. The amount of potential energy in a food is quantified in terms of *calories* (kcals). Carbohydrates and proteins contain about 4 kcal per gram and fats contain 9 kcal per gram. Vitamins and minerals are called *micronutrients* and help us to convert the potential energy from carbohydrates, proteins, and fats into energy the body can use; however, micronutrients do not directly provide energy in the form of calories.

The potential energy stored in food can only be utilized after it has been digested, absorbed, and transported into individual cells. When carbohydrates, fats, and proteins are digested the resulting glucose, fatty acids, and amino acids, respectively, are absorbed from the small intestine and enter into circulation. Once in circulation these molecules can be used immediately or, if caloric intake exceeds energy demands, stored for future use as *glycogen* or as *triglycerides.*

If calories are needed to meet immediate energy demands, glucose, triglycerides, and/or amino acids can be metabolized through oxidative metabolism, except in the case of extremely high-intensity exercise in which anaerobic glycolysis predominates. Oxidative metabolism occurs within the cellular mitochondria, and through a series of complex reactions, glucose, fatty acids, and/or amino acids are used to rephosphorylate adenosine diphosphate (ADP) into *adenosine triphosphate* (ATP). This complex transfer of energy is also referred to as oxidative phosphorylation and is required to convert the energy from food into a currency (ATP) that cells can readily use for biological processes.

When ATP is used it is hydrolyzed. This process releases the energy needed for muscle contraction and many other biological processes. The remaining ADP and Pi must be rephosphorylated to be used again; this happens through the metabolism of carbohydrates, proteins, and fats. This process repeats as long as a cell and/or organism is alive but the rate depends on the energy demand of cell and/or organism. For example exercise, such as running, is a high-energy-demand activity and requires a great increase in the rate at which ATP is produced.

Highly metabolic skeletal muscle cells can rephosphorylate ADP into ATP via the three energy systems: phosphocreatine (PCr), glycolysis, and oxidative phosphorylation. During high-intensity anaerobic exercise the working muscle will preferentially utilize the PCr and glycolytic energy systems because these energy pathways can produce ATP more quickly than oxidative phosphorylation; however, the ability to use these pathways is limited to short, high-intensity bursts of exercise that are less than 90 seconds in length. Repeated utilization of these energy pathways, such as in a football or basketball game, requires frequent rest periods between higher-intensity bouts of exercise. Detailed discussion of these three energy systems is beyond the scope of this book, and for a thorough review of nutrient metabolism refer to the text *Exercise Physiology, Nutrition, Energy, and Human Performance* by McArdle, Katch, and Katch (McArdle et al. 2014) or *Nutrition for Sport and Exercise* by Dunford and Doyle (2015).

Key Points

Energy from foods—specifically from carbohydrates, proteins, and fats—is ultimately converted with the assistance from vitamins and minerals into usable energy the body can use. The three metabolic energy systems (oxidative metabolism, anaerobic glycolysis, and phospho-creatine) harness potential energy stored in macronutrients through a series of oxidation and reduction actions, eventually forming the biologically useful ATP molecule. Optimal functioning of these coordinated systems require proper fueling techniques

Carbohydrates

Carbohydrates are molecules composed of carbon, hydrogen, and oxygen (often abbreviated as CHO). CHO molecules can be short monosaccharides or disaccharides (*simple sugars*) or long polymers (*complex carbohydrates*). Carbohydrates are found in fruits, vegetables, grains, beans, legumes, and even many dairy products. All carbohydrates and sugars, no matter the source, have 4 kcals per gram.

Types of Dietary Carbohydrates

Simple Sugars

Simple sugars are the monosaccharides: glucose, fructose, galactose, and the disaccharides: maltose, sucrose, and lactose. Glucose is the most abundant dietary monosaccharide, although it is usually found in the form of sucrose, which is a glucose molecule attached to a fructose molecule. In the body, glucose is the only carbohydrate found in the blood and the only carbohydrate that is able to be stored for future energy needs. Glucose molecules can be stored within skeletal muscle and liver cells as long glucose polymers called *glycogen*. Glycogen stored within skeletal muscle represents an especially important source of energy for high-intensity exercise. Athletes can be encouraged to think of glycogen as the fuel that allows for high-intensity exercise, and just as gasoline is needed to drive a car, muscles require adequate glycogen stores to be able to perform moderate to high-intensity exercise.

Many foods, such as lasagna, breakfast cereal, and pizza, contain simple sugars as well as complex carbohydrates. Foods which contain naturally occurring simple sugars include fruit and milk, but often simple sugars derived from refined sugar cane, corn, rice, or other sources are added to foods to improve flavor and texture. These sugars are referred to as *added sugar*. Added sugar should be limited within the diet as it provides calories but no vitamins or minerals. Soon, number of grams of added sugars will be indicated on the nutrition facts label.

Recently the World Health Organization (WHO) revised the recommended upper intake of added sugars from 10% of total daily kcals to just 5%; for an individual who consumes 3,000 kcals/day, this represents about 150 kcals, or 9 teaspoons. Physically active individuals can likely consume more than this amount of added sugar without ill effect, but considering the lack of nutrients in most high-sugar products, the WHO recommendations represent a good rule of thumb regardless of physical activity level. Exercise should not be considered a free ticket to consume sugary foods.

Complex Carbohydrates

Complex carbohydrates are long chains of glucose molecules structurally linked together. In the digestive track, prior to absorption and metabolism, these chains must be broken down into individual glucose molecules. Compared to simple carbohydrates, the digestion and absorption of complex carbohydrates requires more time. Many less-processed or unrefined complex carbohydrates also contain fiber, which increases satiety and is beneficial for overall digestive health, but also further slows the digestive process.

Less-processed and unrefined carbohydrates are sometimes referred to as *whole grains*. These types of grains, along with fruits and vegetables, should make up the majority of daily carbohydrate intake because these foods have an abundance of B vitamins, minerals, fiber, and other nutrients not found in highly processed and refined sources. B vitamins are especially important because they are necessary to convert food into energy (ATP).

Less-processed and unrefined whole grain complex carbohydrates include the following:

- Whole wheat breads/bagels/crackers (WHOLE wheat listed as first ingredient)
- Whole wheat tortillas
- Brown rice
- Whole wheat pasta
- Beans
- 100% whole grain cereals (Wheaties, Cheerios, Shredded Wheat)
- Oatmeal (not the instant packets)
- Sweet potatoes
- Corn
- Exotic grains (quinoa, bulgur, millet, rye, buckwheat, barley, and wheat germ)

Processed or refined carbohydrates can still be considered complex since the molecular structure consists of polymers. Examples of refined complex carbohydrates include foods such as white pasta, white flour tortillas, white rice, French fries, crackers, cookies, cereal bars, pancakes, and breads not listing WHOLE wheat as the first ingredient. Compared to whole or less processed sources, refined carbohydrates tend to have less vitamins, minerals, protein, and fiber, and they often have more added sugars and sodium. Whole grains are nutritionally superior, and the majority of complex carbohydrates should be consumed in this form, along with starchy vegetables and legumes.

Fiber

Fiber is a type of complex carbohydrate humans cannot digest; therefore, fiber does not provide any calories (for cows it is another story). Many unprocessed plant-based foods contain dietary fiber which can be further classified as *soluble fiber* or *insoluble fiber*. Both types are important to include in the diet as each provides unique health benefits.

Fiber is important for the following reasons:
- Satiety (feeling full)
- Healthy cholesterol levels
- Healthy digestive system
- Healthy body weight

Some foods contain both soluble and insoluble fibers, but in general whole fruits (not juice), beans, and oatmeal are packed with soluble fiber, whereas vegetables and other unrefined grains contain primarily insoluble fiber. Daily fiber recommendations are approximately 25 g/day for a 2,000 kcal/day diet. Daily fiber intake should increase as caloric content of the diet increases; for example, an athlete who consumes 3,000 kcal/day should aim for 35 g of fiber each day. Good wholefood sources of fiber are listed in Table 1.1.

Absorption, Metabolism, and Storage of Dietary Carbohydrate

Dietary carbohydrates are only available as energy after being completely digested and absorbed from the small intestine. All carbohydrates, no matter the source, are eventually broken down into monosaccharides (glucose, fructose, and galactose) prior to absorption. After absorption, monosaccharides are transported to the liver where galactose and fructose molecules are converted into glucose. Glucose is then transported to the rest of the body via the circulatory system where it is available for cellular uptake and utilized for ATP production, stored as glycogen, or converted into triglycerides and stored within the adipose.

The fate of glucose, once it has been transported to the liver, is dependent upon the body's energy balance, that is how much energy the body requires compared with what is being consumed, as well as daily carbohydrate consumption. If more carbohydrate has been consumed than immediately needed for the production of ATP, excess can be stored as glycogen within the liver and muscle cells. As mentioned previously,

Table 1.1 Foods naturally high in fiber as well as grams of fiber per serving

Source	Fiber per serving (g)
Apples	4.5 g per medium fruit
Bananas	3.1 g per medium fruit
Dry oatmeal	4.0 g per ½ cup
Black beans	10 g per ½ cup
Refried beans	6 g per ½ cup
Whole wheat bread	Varies depending on brand 1–4 g
Almonds	3.5 g per 1 oz
Berries	3 g per 1 cup
Broccoli	4 g per ½ cup raw
Soy nuts	3.5 g per ¼ cup

glycogen is a polysaccharide made of multiple glucose molecules linked together. This source of energy can be drawn upon when energy intake does not meet energy demand. For example, energy demand of the working muscle can be met through the breakdown and metabolism of intracellular muscle glycogen stores and during periods of fasting or low blood glucose, liver glycogen stores can be broken down into glucose and released into the blood.

The central nervous system (CNS), which includes the brain, requires and draws upon the glucose in the blood to meet energy needs and function. When blood glucose levels decrease, as can happen when liver glycogen is depleted, motivation and the ability to think and react quickly are diminished. Maintaining blood glucose levels above 70 mg/dL is important because if blood glucose becomes too low, symptoms of hypoglycemia may appear and the ability to concentrate dwindles. Fueling the brain with adequate glucose is important for optimal performance in sports that involve decision-making, tactics, focus, and concentration (i.e., all sports). The brain also develops and sends the message about how and where to move the rest of the body, and if adequate carbohydrate is not available, this message would not be relayed properly.

Unlike the CNS, most other cells in the body can metabolize fat and amino acids in addition to glucose. At rest, fat is the primary source of energy used to meet energy demand. But when energy demand is high, such as during exercise, glycogen stored within the contracting muscle will provide ATP at a faster rate and will be the preferred fuel source. As such, intramuscular glycogen stores are a very important source of energy during high-intensity exercise. However, glycogen stores are limited and can be depleted when exercise is very intense and lasts longer than 90 to 120 minutes. When stores within the muscle are depleted athletic performance suffers because glycogen is one of the primary fuels required for maximal force and power production. Glycogen depletion during exercise cannot be completely avoided, but beginning exercise with optimal stores can delay the onset of depletion-induced fatigue.

Consuming inadequate carbohydrate leads to glycogen depletion which causes the following:
- Earlier signs of physical and mental fatigue
- Reduced power output and force production
- Decreased aerobic and anaerobic performance
- Slower recovery between training sessions
- Generally feeling lousy

Glycogen stores can be optimally stocked through the following practices:
- Adequate daily caloric intake
- Consuming a moderate to high carbohydrate diet (45 to 65 percent of daily kcal intake, depending on training intensity, frequency, and duration)
- Consuming additional carbohydrates on very intense or long training/competition days
- Consuming carbohydrate-containing foods within 30 minutes after intense training/competition

Consuming carbohydrates in amounts above and beyond what can be utilized for energy production or stored as glycogen does not reap additional benefits. Once liver and muscle glycogen stores are fully stocked (think of a full tank of gas), additional glucose is converted into triglycerides and stored within adipocytes (fat cells).

Daily Carbohydrate Needs

Daily carbohydrate requirements are based on body weight, body composition, and training demands including exercise frequency, duration, and intensity. For a general estimation, the values in Table 1.2 can be used to approximate daily carbohydrate needs based on training duration and nature of the sport.

To use Table 1.2, the athlete's body weight in kilograms must be known; calculate this by dividing his or her weight in pounds by 2.2. Once weight in kilograms has been calculated, multiply this value by the activity factor that is most appropriate for the athlete (based on sport and training duration). The range of values within Table 1.2 allows for a more precise estimation; the lower end of the range should be used

Table 1.2 Approximate daily carbohydrate needs based on training duration and nature of the sport. Values are given in grams per kilogram of body weight (g/kg/bw)

	Aerobic Endurance Sports	Anaerobic/ Aerobic Sports	Anaerobic Power Sports
Sporting types and examples	Distance running, cycling, cross-country skiing, swimming, rowing, triathlon	Soccer, basketball, lacrosse, singles tennis, running events <1,600 meters	American football, rugby, gymnastics, hockey, volleyball, downhill skiing, track and field events, resistance training
Exercise/practice duration within a 24-hour period	*Daily CHO needs (assumes continuous activity)*	*Daily CHO needs (assumes stop and go activity)*	*Daily CHO needs (assumes stop and go activity)*
60 min/day	5–7	5	5
60–90 min/day	6–8	5–7	5–7
90–120 min/day	7–9	6–8	5–7
2–3 hours/day	7–10	7–9	6–8
3–4 hours/day	8–12	8–10	6–8
>4 hours/day	>10	>9	>8

when training is not quite as long or intense or if there is generally a lot of stop and go throughout a practice session. The upper end of the range is for harder, longer training days and/or continuous movement. Intensity of training can alter carbohydrate needs dramatically and as exercise intensity increases, total energy expenditure increases and a greater percentage of that energy demand is met through the metabolism of carbohydrate (as opposed to fat which is utilized at lower exercise intensities and at rest).

An example calculation for a 16-year-old American football player who practices for 2½ hours each day (0:45 morning weight session; 1:45 afternoon practice):
- Weight in pounds = 160 lbs
- Weight in kilogram = 160/2.2 = 72.7 kg
- Using Table 1.2, the appropriate range of carbohydrate intake is approximately 6 to 8 g/kg/day
- Lower daily recommended CHO intake: Multiply body weight in kilogram by 6
  - 72.7 × 6 = 436 g CHO per day (1,745 kcals/day)
- Upper daily recommended CHO intake: Multiply body weight in kilogram by 8
  - 72.7 × 8 = 582 g CHO per day (2,326 kcals/day)

Timing of Carbohydrate Intake

When carbohydrates are eaten is as important as *total amount* of carbohydrates eaten. The following provides general guidelines for timing of carbohydrate consumption.

Before exercise: A carbohydrate-rich snack should be eaten 30 to 60 minutes prior to exercise if it has been more than 3 or 4 hours since the last meal. Low blood sugar is somewhat more likely 3 to 4 hours postprandial (after eating) and can lead to low energy levels and lack of focus. Having an athlete consume an appropriate snack of about 30 to 50 g of carbohydrate (about 120 to 200 kcals) that is low in fat and fiber can help prevent low blood glucose levels. Refer to Table 1.3 for carbohydrate content of specific foods. Fatty foods as well as those high in fiber and/or protein should be avoided immediately prior to exercise because they delay digestion and absorption which increases likelihood of gastrointestinal (GI) distress. However, consuming a *small* amount of protein (about 10 g) 30 minutes prior to exercise may be beneficial as recent research indicates a positive performance and recovery effect, especially in the case of resistance training.

During exercise: Consuming carbohydrate during exercise can help maintain physical and mental performance and motivation. Sports drink, such as Gatorade, is a popular option for exercise longer than an hour since these beverages also serve to meet fluid and electrolyte needs with minimal risk of stomach upset. The amount of sports drink needed depends on duration and intensity of activity, but 16 to 24 ounces per hour is a rough estimate. For exercise less than an hour, water is typically sufficient unless the athlete is exercising in extremely hot weather, in which case sports drink can be used as a means to replace lost electrolytes. Also of note, recent research indicates that consuming a *small* amount of protein (about 5 g per hour) in addition to carbohydrate *during* exercise *may* elicit greater benefits than carbohydrate alone. If a training session or competition lasts longer than 1 hour, sport gels or gummy candies (Shot Blocks) are also an option, but these are best taken with water and not sports drink as the ingestion of too many simple sugars slows intestinal absorption. Always experiment with new foods and fluids during training *not* during a race or competition.

After exercise: The body recovers more quickly when carbohydrates and protein are eaten shortly after a training session or competition. A carbohydrate-rich snack should be eaten within 60 minutes postexercise, followed by a carbohydrate-rich meal within 2 hours. This practice becomes more important as exercise duration, intensity, and frequency increases with athletic ability and maturity. Evidence from multiple researchers clearly shows that recovery is further facilitated when 10 to 20 g of protein is consumed in addition to carbohydrate. *A general recommendation for athletes who exercise at a moderate to high intensity for at least 60 minutes each day: Consume about 50 g of carbohydrate and 10 to 20 g of protein within 30 to 60 minutes postexercise; repeat within 90 minutes if a meal is not available.* Sources of carbohydrate- and protein-containing foods can be found in Table 1.3.

Carbohydrates for Endurance Athletes

Athletes participating in endurance sports such as cross-country skiing and running, swimming, triathlon, and cycling have unique nutritional

Table 1.3 Sources of convenient pre- and postexercise carbohydrates and proteins

Food	Carbohydrate (g)	Protein (g)
1 slice whole grain bread*	22–25	2–5
1 cup Wheaties	30	3
1 medium-sized banana	22–25	2
1 cup low-fat chocolate milk	20–26	8
¼ cup raisins	29	1
1 cup cooked pasta	36	8
1 medium baked potato	35–40	4
1 cup cooked brown rice	46	4
1 cup fruited low-fat yogurt (not "Greek")*	40–50	8–12
1 bagel (from a bagel shop)*	55–65	5–10
1 slice of veggie pizza (not deep dish)*	30–40	8–12
1 bean and cheese burrito (fast food)*	70–80	10–20
½ cup pinto beans	22	8
1 Cliff bar	45	5–10

* Approximate, actual grams depends on brand and store.

needs. These sports generally require greater caloric and carbohydrate intake because movement is constant (rather than stop and go as is the case in most anaerobic team sports). Optimal training and performance for continuous aerobic exercise requires optimal glycogen stores.

Caloric expenditure associated with moderate- to high-intensity aerobic exercise can be anywhere between 500 and 1,000+ kcals/per hour. If the energy expended during training is not replaced, over time an athlete may experience the following:

- Unintentional weight loss
- Decreased performance
- Increased fatigue during and after training
- Increased risk of injury
- Injuries that will not heal
- Increased number of colds/illness
- Slower recovery between workouts
- Poor sleep
- Achy muscles

To avoid these symptoms, it is important to begin training sessions with fully stocked glycogen stores and replenish stores soon after training. Eating carbohydrate-rich foods within an hour of training helps to restore muscle glycogen levels. After this 60-minute window glycogen replenishment is slowed, resulting in delayed recovery. This is particularly relevant to athletes who have less than 24 hours to recover before their next training session.

Carbohydrate Loading.   Carbo-loading is a practice used by many athletes the night before a big event. While technically carbohydrate loading is a 3-day-plus regimented protocol used to increase the glycogen storage capacity of the muscles, eating carbohydrate-rich meals the evening before a big event or training session is a common practice among many athletes. The meal of choice is generally pasta but any carbohydrate source (potatoes, rice, and bread) is just as effective. Although a high-carbohydrate dinner is a good pre-event meal, overeating is not necessary and may cause bloating and GI distress. Carbo-loading is a useful practice for endurance events lasting over 90 minutes (such as marathons), but is not generally necessary or helpful for events <90 minutes in length. Assuming the athlete is consuming adequate kcals and carbohydrates on a daily basis, it is likely that adequate glycogen stores will be available if an athlete eats the usual-sized dinner and breakfast.

Key Points

Adequate carbohydrate intake is essential for optimal athletic performance and recovery. Glucose is the primary fuel source for the CNS as well as high intensity muscle contraction. Athletes should focus on fruits, vegetables, legumes, whole grains, and milk and yogurt as their primary sources of dietary carbohydrates and should limit the intake of added sugars and refined grains. Daily carbohydrate needs are dependent on body weight, exercise intensity and duration, and body weight goals. In general endurance athletes have higher needs than team or power sport athletes. All athletes must be mindful of consuming adequate carbohydrates before and after exercise and, if exercise duration is >60 minutes, during exercise.

Protein

Proteins are complex molecules made from unique combinations and configurations of the 20 *amino acids*. Adequate dietary protein is required for muscle growth and muscle maintenance but is also essential for healthy hair, skin, tendons, ligaments, bones, blood, and many other functions essential to life. Unlike carbohydrate and fat, protein is generally not a primary fuel source because every protein in the body serves a role and, if oxidized for energy, will need to be resynthesized later. This is also true of circulating individual amino acids; amino acids used for energy during exercise will no longer be available to make needed proteins, such as those required for tissue repair or muscle growth.

Dietary proteins have 4 kcals per gram and are found in many food sources. Meat, fish, dairy, nuts, and legumes are rich sources of protein. Dietary proteins are broken down into amino acids in the small intestine. Individual amino acids can then be absorbed and transported to the liver, eventually becoming part of the circulating amino acid pool. This pool of free amino acids exists in circulation as well as in the liver and can be drawn from to make needed proteins. The body can build all the proteins required to survive and thrive, but to do so, adequate amounts of all the 20 different amino acids must be available. The liver can even *make* some of these amino acids (*nonessential amino acids*), but others must come from protein-containing foods (*essential amino acids*).

While the liver can make some amino acids (nonessential and conditionally essential amino acids), it cannot make essential amino acids and, in some cases, cannot make adequate amounts of conditionally essential amino acids. Therefore, these amino acids must be obtained through the diet. Protein sources that contain all nine essential amino acids, in adequate quantities, are considered complete proteins and include all animal and soy proteins. Incomplete protein sources *may* contain all nine essential amino acids but not in sufficient quantities. All non–animal-based proteins, with the exception of soy, are incomplete. Not all incomplete proteins lack the same essential amino acid(s). For example, grains, nuts, and seeds lack in the essential amino acid lysine, but beans and legumes are rich in lysine; therefore, by combining two incomplete proteins, such as rice and beans or peanut butter and bread, it is possible to obtain all essential amino acids.

The body's ability to synthesize new proteins is dependent upon supply and demand. Supply refers to adequate number and type of amino acids within the pool and demand refers to the need to build or repair something within the body. For optimal protein synthesis the circulating amino acid pool (supply) should be filled several times throughout the day; this is accomplished by consuming foods with moderate to high amounts of protein. However, if one wishes to hypertrophy muscle it is also essential to increase demand. Therefore, it is essential to resistance train *in addition* to eating protein. Furthermore, the intensity of resistance training must continually provide sufficient overload for the adaptation and hypertrophy process to continue. In the case of endurance exercise, athletes who train at moderate to high intensities need to continually replenish the amino acid pool in order to make up for any amino acids that are oxidized during exercise as well as repair any damaged tissues. As always, more is not necessarily better. In the event that amino acid capacity within the pool has been reached (about 1.5 to 2.5 g/kg/bw daily), excess will be oxidized for energy, converted into glucose or, more likely, converted and stored as adipose (fat).

Daily Protein Needs

The approximate amount of protein the body needs for repair and growth depends on muscle mass, demands placed on the body, and body composition/weight goals. Protein needs especially increase for athletes who are starting to lift weights or are engaging in very high-intensity training because the body requires additional amino acids as a backup fuel source and to build muscle mass. Sedentary adults need as little as 1 g/kg of body weight, but growing athletes should aim for about 1.5 to 2.5 g/kg of body weight. More than this amount is not beneficial because synthesis of new proteins cannot keep pace with protein intake. In the event protein intake exceeds protein synthesis, additional amino acids will be oxidized, converted to glucose and stored as glycogen, or converted to adipose and stored as fat. Too much dietary protein can also crowd out needed carbohydrates and fats.

Other factors that can increase protein requirements include the following:
- Increases in fat-free mass
- Low dietary intake of carbohydrates
- Low total caloric intake
- Relatively low bioavailability of protein sources (most plant proteins)
- Increases in exercise training, frequency, intensity, and duration
- Acute or chronic injuries and any existing disease state

Dietary protein is used most efficiently for protein synthesis when we eat small, frequent protein-containing meals and snacks throughout the day. If protein intake exceeds 30 g at a time, protein synthesis cannot keep pace and a portion of the ingested amino acids will not be used for new protein synthesis, rather some of these amino acids will be oxidized or converted to glucose or fat and stored. *A general recommendation for protein intake is to consume 20 to 30 g of protein four to seven plus times throughout the day (depending on your specific caloric and protein needs). A realistic way to achieve this is to aim for 20 to 30 g of protein at each meal and about 5 to 10 g at each snack.* Table 1.4 gives examples of protein-containing foods.

Table 1.4 Protein content and serving size of various foods

Food	Serving Size	Amount of Protein (g)
Chicken breast	3 oz	27
Tuna (in water)	1 can	41
Hamburger	3 oz	22
Cottage cheese	½ cup	14
Yogurt (fruited)	6 oz.	6
Greek yogurt (fruited)	6 oz	14
Peanut butter	2 tbsp	8
Nuts	1 oz	6
Cheese	1 oz	7
Beans	½ cup	8
Tofu (firm)	½ cup	10
Egg	1 white + 1 yolk	6
Milk	8 oz (1 cup)	8
Pasta	½ cup uncooked	8

Many athletes consume protein and amino acid shakes and bars in an effort to improve strength and increase rate of hypertrophy, but it is not necessary to use these expensive products. There is no research to suggest that protein or amino acid supplements improve performance to a greater degree than protein in real food nor are they needed for athletes to meet their protein needs. It is known that the body utilizes foods that naturally contain protein just as well (and sometimes better) as expensive protein or amino acid supplements. However, protein bars and shakes may be convenient and useful when meat and dairy are not available or cannot be kept cold. These products will be discussed further in the chapter on dietary supplements.

Key Points

Athletes have greater protein needs than their nonathletic peers; however, increased needs can be met by consuming a variety of protein-containing foods including meat, eggs, fish, dairy, legumes, nuts, seeds, and soy. Because the body cannot store protein for future use, athletes should consume moderate amounts of protein consistently throughout the day. Consuming a small amount of protein within 60 minutes of, or during, exercise may enhance performance and there is consistent evidence to support the ergogenic benefits of high-quality protein consumption in the postexercise period.

Fats

Dietary fat and body fat are part of a group of molecules called *lipids*. *Body fat* refers to the triglycerides stored in *adipose* cells. Adipose cells make up the subcutaneous and visceral fat tissues which serve to insulate the body and protect the internal organs. If needed, these triglyceride stores can be broken down, released into circulation, and used by other cells as a source of energy (ATP). Fats stored within muscle cells are called *intramuscular triglycerides*. These triglycerides are a convenient source of energy for the muscle cell during aerobic exercise. After exercise, fats in circulation will be preferentially used to restore muscle triglyceride levels (as opposed to being stored as subcutaneous or visceral fat).

At 9 kcals per gram, fat is the most energy dense of the macronutrients. Dietary fats serve many important roles. Specifically, dietary fat is essential for the absorption of fat-soluble vitamins A, D, E, and K. The consumption of fat is also required for healthy cell membranes, the creation of certain steroid hormones such as testosterone, and even regulation of the inflammatory process. Omega-3 fatty acids in particular play important roles in muscle recovery, arterial health, and reduction of the inflammatory response. Both dietary and body fats act as an important source of energy at rest and during low- to moderate-intensity exercise.

Fat is the body's fuel of choice for lower-intensity exercise and many other activities such as walking, sitting, Internet surfing, even rest intervals between sets at the gym. The body can also rely on a mix of fat, glycogen, and blood glucose to meet energy needs during low- to moderate-intensity exercise; however, as exercise intensity begins to increase, the muscle cells begin to rely on stored muscle glycogen and blood glucose to a greater extent. Although glycogen and glucose can provide ATP more quickly than fats, eventually glycogen stores within specific muscle groups dwindle and exercise intensity must decrease because ATP demands cannot be met as quickly when there is an increased reliance on fat as the primary energy substrate. As an athlete becomes more aerobically fit, the ability to utilize fat for the production of ATP at rest and during low to moderate exercise intensities is enhanced. This is beneficial because using fat instead of glycogen allows the athlete to exercise longer and at a higher intensity before becoming glycogen depleted.

Types of Dietary Fat

There are three primary categories of dietary triglycerides (fats): *saturated fats, unsaturated fats, and trans fats.* This classification is based on molecular structure, specifically, the number and position of carbon double bonds.

Trans-fatty acids (*Trans* fats)

Unprocessed or minimally processed foods contain no or negligible amounts of *trans* fats. This is true for even very high-fat foods such as butter, lard, and vegetable oils. Food scientists, however, learned the process of partial hydrogenation in order to create what is commonly known as a *trans* fat.

These chemically altered fats are being phased out of all aspects of the food industry and will no longer be available for home or commercial frying, baking, or added to processed food products because it is now known that consumption of *trans* fats is strongly associated with decreases in high-density lipoproteins (HDL or good cholesterol) and increases in low-density lipoproteins (LDL or bad cholesterol). Reductions in HDL and increases in LDL set the stage for atherosclerosis and poor arterial function; therefore, until these fats are completely eliminated from the marketplace, avoid *trans* fats all together. If the list of ingredients contains *partially hydrogenated oil* then there are *trans* fats in the product even if the label lists 0 g. Avoid these products since no amount of trans fat provides any benefit and any amount may be detrimental to cardiovascular health.

Saturated fatty acids (Saturated fats)

Saturated fats are found in animal products, chocolate (cocoa butter), coconut oil, palm oil, and many processed and/or packaged foods. Previously, diets high in saturated fat have been associated with an increased risk of cardiovascular disease and other chronic health conditions; currently some of those finding and associations are being challenged. For now it is safe to say that the link between saturated fat intake and cardiovascular health is not as cut and dry as was once thought, and based on available evidence, some dietary saturated fat is not detrimental to overall health. However, this is not a free ticket to bacon heaven, as red and processed meats are still thought to increase risk for chronic diseases. Additionally, too much saturated fat can crowd out other more beneficial dietary fats. A reasonable recommendation for dietary saturated fat is 10 to 15 percent of daily kcal intake. Putting this into context, an athlete who eats 3,000 kcals/day should consume no more than about 30 to 35 g of saturated fat daily. Grams of saturated fat as well as percent of recommended daily intake of saturated fat (based on a 2,000 kcal/day intake) can be found on the nutrition facts label. Keep in mind, however, that these values are based on a single serving.

Foods high in saturated fat:
- Butter (1 tablespoon has 12 g of fat and 8 g of saturated fat)
- Sour cream

- Cheese
- Whole milk and ice cream
- Beef, pork, lamb
- Chicken with the skin
- Palm oil and coconut oil (found in many packaged foods)
- Chocolate
- Most pastries and desserts

Unsaturated fatty acids (Unsaturated Fats)

Unsaturated fats are found in varying amounts in both animal and plant products. Foods especially high in unsaturated fats include extracted fish and vegetable oils, nuts, avocado, and seeds. Unsaturated fats can be further categorized as monounsaturated or polyunsaturated, and poly- unsaturated fats are classified as either omega-3 or omega-6. Similar to saturated fats, all classification is based on fatty acid structure and specifi- cally the number and location of carbon double bonds.

Dietary fats that contain appreciable amounts of omega-3 fatty acids, such as canola oil, fish oils, and the oils from certain nuts and seeds, may prevent cardiovascular disease, reduce inflammation throughout the body, and promote recovery of injured tissues. Evidence for the beneficial effects of omega-3 fatty acid consumption is strong and research findings have shown that consuming adequate omega-3 fatty acids reduces exercise-in- duced inflammation and muscle damage as well as inflammation due to muscle injury. Omega-3 fatty acids potentially have a variety of health ben- efits but are especially scarce in the typical American diet. Some evidence suggests that the ratio of omega-6:omega-3 fatty acids is important for con- trolling the body's inflammation process and the American diet is too rich in omega-6 fatty acids (such as from soybean and safflower oils) and lacking in omega-3s. A diet rich in monounsaturated fats, moderate in omega-6 polyunsaturated fats, and includes at least 3 g/day of omega-3 polyunsatu- rated fats likely supports long-term health as well as athletic performance.

Foods high in unsaturated fats:
- Olive oil (monounsaturated fat)
- Canola oil (polyunsaturated omega-6, omega-3, and monounsaturated fats)

- Avocados (monounsaturated fat)
- Sesame oil (polyunsaturated omega-6, omega-3, and monounsaturated fats)
- Safflower oil (polyunsaturated omega-6 and monounsaturated fats)
- Fatty fish (tuna, salmon, sardines) (omega-3 fats)
- Nuts and seeds (polyunsaturated omega-3 and monounsaturated fats)
- Flax seeds (ground) and walnuts (omega-3 fats)

Cholesterol

Unlike triglycerides, cholesterol has a ring-like molecular structure and is classified as a sterol. Cholesterol is made endogenously by the liver and is an important component of cell membranes as well as a precursor for certain hormones such as estrogen and testosterone. Cholesterol can be obtained from dietary sources but since the liver makes adequate amounts, consuming cholesterol is not necessary. In fact, for certain individuals, too much dietary cholesterol can increase the amount of cholesterol in the blood which may increase risk for cardiovascular disease. However, blood cholesterol levels are negatively influenced to a greater degree by excessive refined carbohydrate, saturated fat, and *trans* fat intake as opposed to actual cholesterol intake. In general foods that are high in cholesterol include egg yolks, fatty cuts of meat, full-fat dairy products, organ meat, and some types of shellfish. Plant-based foods contain no cholesterol.

Estimating Daily Fat Needs and Sources of Dietary Fats

Athletes should consume roughly 20 to 35 percent of daily calories from fat. This amount ensures optimal health and leaves room for adequate intake of carbohydrate and protein. Putting this range into perspective, if an athlete eats about 3,000 kcals a day, about 600 to 1,000 kcals/day (or about 70 to 110 g/day) should come from fat. Another general guideline for fat intake is the estimate of 1 to 2 g per kilogram of body weight each day. Since this is a rather large range, it is best to first calculate carbohydrate and protein needs then estimate the amount of fat needed based on remaining required daily caloric intake. In general, the lower end of the range is for athletes with lower kcal demands and the higher end is appropriate for athletes with higher kcal demands.

Some of the more obvious sources of fat, such as butter and plant oils, can be easily identified; however, often the majority of dietary fat does not come from the fat *added* to our food, rather it comes from meats, cheese, milk, yogurt, pizza, cakes, cookies, crackers, chips, and bars. Even breads and grains have a small amount of fat. As a rule of thumb choose healthy fats such as almonds, walnuts, flax, nut butters, seeds, healthy oils, and avocado-based dips. Table 1.5 details the fat content of common foods, also listed is the *type* of fat.

Table 1.5 Fat content in grams (g) and type of fat in common foods

Food	Serving Size	Total Fat (g)	Saturated (g)	Unsaturated (g)
Deep dish pepperoni pizza	1 slice	25	12	13
Thin crust veggie pizza	1 slice	9	4	5
French fries	1 medium order	15	3	12
Baked potato	1 medium	0.5	0.1	0.4
Fish sticks	4 sticks	11	3	8
Grilled salmon	3 oz	7	1	6
Ice cream	½ cup	8	5	3
Frozen yogurt	½ cup	3	1.5	1.5
Lasagna	1 restaurant serving	33	15	18
Pasta with marinara sauce	1 cup pasta and ½ cup sauce	4	1	3
Beef burrito with sour cream	1 burrito with 2 tbsp sour cream	44	17	27
Bean and cheese burrito with avocado	1 burrito with ⅓ avocado	16	5	11
Blueberry muffin	1 large muffin	19	3.5	15.5
Blueberry bagel	1 large bagel	1.5	0	1.5
Whole chocolate milk	1 cup	9	6	3
1% chocolate milk	1 cup	3	1.5	1.5
Movie theater popcorn	1 medium	25	22	3
Air-popped popcorn	5 cups	1	0	1
Almonds	1 oz	14	1	13

Key Points

Dietary and body fats serve a variety of essential functions and represent a source of energy at rest and during low intensity exercise. Because fats are energy dense, it is important to moderate intake. Type of fat consumed is also important, unsaturated fats including avocado, nuts and seeds, olive oil, and fish should represent the majority of fat intake. Saturated fats found in dairy foods are not as unhealthful as previously thought, though athletes should limit their intake of red and processed meats.

Micronutrients

Vitamins and minerals are called *micronutrients*. Micronutrients have many essential functions including building and maintaining bone, oxygen delivery to the cells, proper immune function, energy production during rest and exercise, and protecting the cells from oxidative stress. There are 13 known vitamins and at least 16 minerals that are considered essential for life; other minerals such as nickel, silicon, vanadium, and cobalt are also thought to be essential but only in extremely small quantities. Choline is also an essential nutrient, although sometimes classified as a vitamin, it is technically not a vitamin nor a mineral. Micronutrients, unlike macronutrients, are required in rather small quantities and do not provide energy (calories).

In general whole, unprocessed foods will have more vitamins and minerals than processed and packaged foods. The exception to this generalization is if the processed food product has been *fortified* or *enriched*. Enrichment refers to when a food, through processing, has been stripped of some of the original nutritional value and some of the lost vitamins and minerals are then added back. Enrichment of refined wheat flour is a common example. *Fortified* foods contain added nutrients that were never present prior to processing. Common fortified foods include breakfast cereals, breakfast cereal bars, sports bars, and many beverages. Fortified wholegrain cereals and milk are an important source of vitamins, minerals, carbohydrates, fiber, and even protein but there are also many fortified foods that are low-fiber and high-sugar and provide little nutritional benefit other than their added vitamins and minerals—avoid these types of products.

In almost all cases micronutrient needs can be met through the consumption of *whole foods* like fruits, vegetables, whole grains, nuts, seeds, beans, and low-fat sources of dairy and meat. Taking a multivitamin and mineral supplement is not harmful; it may also help to provide peace of mind and in some instances may prevent or amend specific deficiencies in susceptible individuals, *but* it is important to not rely on a supplement to make up for a nutrient-poor diet. See Chapter 5 on more details of multivitamin supplementation.

Micronutrients for Energy Metabolism and Production

In order to produce the ATP needed for muscle contraction and other essential processes, macronutrients, namely carbohydrates and fat, must be metabolized. Metabolic processes occur within all cells of the body and require not only available substrate (macronutrients) but also a variety of vitamins and minerals. In fact, in a classic nutrition study, animals that were fed pure carbohydrates, proteins, and fats but with no vitamins and minerals died fairly quickly due to the inability to utilize the macronutrients that were consumed! Table 1.6 highlights the vitamins and minerals

Table 1.6 Micronutrients needed for the metabolism of macronutrients and sources

Micronutrients Needed for ATP Production	Good Dietary Sources
Thiamine (B$_1$)	• Lean cuts of pork and ham • Whole grains • Fortified breakfast cereals • Enriched grains • Beans and legumes
Riboflavin (B$_2$)	• Beef and chicken liver • Fortified breakfast cereals • Milk • Eggs • Almonds

Micronutrients Needed for ATP Production	Good Dietary Sources
Niacin (B_3)	• Chicken • Turkey • Salmon • Tuna • Fortified cereals • Peanut butter
B6	• All bran • Chicken (light meat) • Garbanzo beans • Lean beef • Lean pork • Baked potato (with skin)
B_{12} (Cobalamin)	• Clams • Crab • Fortified cereals • Sardines • Salmon • Beef • Tuna • Yogurt
Pantothenic acid	• Beef and chicken liver • Sunflower seeds • Mushrooms • Yogurt • Turkey and chicken (dark meat)
Choline (not actually a vitamin)	• Eggs • Beef liver • Beef • Cauliflower (cooked)
Chromium	• Mushrooms • Prunes • DARK chocolate • Nuts • Asparagus

essential for macronutrients to be metabolized into ATP as well as good dietary sources of each micronutrient.

Micronutrients for Red Blood Cell Production and Oxygen Delivery

Red blood cells (hemoglobin) transport oxygen to the cells of the body via the circulatory system. Adequate oxygen delivery to the cells of the working musculature is extremely important for aerobic metabolism as well as recovery between bouts of intense anaerobic exercise. Iron is an essential mineral that helps to form red blood cells that carry oxygen to the working muscles. If adequate amounts of iron are not available, new red blood cells cannot be made. The resultant decrease in red blood cell count is known as *iron deficiency anemia, or anemia.* Anemia can dramatically impair sport performance because any drop in red blood cell count impairs oxygen delivery. See Chapter 5 for more specifics on iron supplementation. Table 1.7 highlights the vitamins and minerals essential for red blood cell production as well as good dietary sources of each micronutrient.

Micronutrients for Cell Protection and Immunity

Some vitamins and minerals act as intracellular and intra-arterial *antioxidants.* These nutrients play a critical role in preventing oxidative damage to the cells and support overall immune function. High doses of anti-oxidant supplements are not required to combat oxidative stress; in fact research findings suggest that mega doses of antioxidants can actually *increase* oxidative stress and cause damage to the cells. Beware of antioxidant supplements or foods that are highly fortified (over 100 percent of the Dietary Reference Intakes, or DRI's), as these may have a *pro-oxidative* effect. The best source of antioxidants is in the form of food, as no upper level of intake of fruits and vegetables has been associated with the negative pro-oxidative effects found with excessive consumption of antioxidant supplements. Table 1.8 highlights vitamins and minerals essential for cell protection and immunity as well as good dietary sources of these important antioxidants.

Table 1.7 Micronutrients essential for adequate production of healthy red blood cells and sources

Micronutrients Required for Red Blood Cell Production	Good Dietary Sources
Iron (absorption is enhanced by vitamin C and impaired by calcium)	• Clams • Oysters • Lentils • Lean beef • Lean chicken • Fish • Spinach • Fortified breakfast cereals
Zinc (absorbed best from animal products, vegetarians should choose a cereal that is fortified with zinc)	• Oysters (raw) • Fortified breakfast cereals • Crab • Lean beef • Pork • Lamb
Copper	• Oysters • Lobster • Mushrooms • Pork • Cashews • Garbanzo beans • Baked potato (with skin) • Spinach
Folate (folic acid); also prevents neural tube defects	• Enriched wheat products (such as enriched bagels, bread, pasta—anything that lists enriched wheat flour as an ingredient) • Lentils • Spinach • Broccoli • Fortified cereals • Pinto beans
B^{12} (deficiency is called pernicious anemia; also activates folate into its active form); vegetarians and vegans should choose a B^{12}-fortified cereal or soymilk	• Clams • Crab • Beef • Salmon • Yogurt • Fortified cereals and soymilks

Table 1.8 Vitamins and minerals that protect cells from oxidative damage and dietary sources

Micronutrient Antioxidants and Supporter of Immune System	Good Dietary Sources
Vitamin E	• Sunflower seeds • Nuts • Avocado • Peanuts and peanut butter • Canola oil • Spinach • Tomato sauces and ketchup
Vitamin C (antioxidant properties and supports immune system)	• Berries • Peppers • Citrus fruits • Strawberries • Kiwi fruit
Vitamin A (also required for healthy vision; deadly toxic in large quantities; acts as a pro-oxidant in quantities over the DRI—do NOT supplement with vitamin A)	• Animal liver contains very high amounts (too much is toxic; polar explorers in the 1800s died of toxicity due to consumption of polar bear liver). • Recommend intake via nontoxic β-carotene sources
β-Carotene (plant-based precursor or provitamin to vitamin A, converted into active vitamin A in the small intestine; *not toxic in large quantities*; also part of the phytochemical class of carotenoids)	• Pumpkin • Sweet potato (with skin) • Spinach • Kale • Carrots • Cantaloupe • Spinach
Selenium	• Halibut • Tuna • Nuts • Turkey • Whole grains • Pork
Zinc (absorbed best from animal products; vegetarians should choose a cereal that is fortified with zinc; antioxidant properties and supports immune system)	• Oysters (raw) • Fortified breakfast cereals • Crab • Lean beef • Pork • Lamb

Bone Health

Many vitamins and minerals play an active role in increasing bone density, promoting bone growth, and strengthening the connective tissue. Bone is a very dynamic tissue and can increase or decrease in density in accordance with the amount of overload placed on it as well as dietary intake of the building blocks essential for bone development. Table 1.9 highlights all the vitamins and minerals required for optimal bone development and outlines dietary sources rich in these important nutrients. In addition it should be noted that adequate protein intake is also essential

Table1.9 Vitamins and minerals essential for bone growth and mineralization and dietary sources

Vitamins and Minerals for Bone Development	Good Dietary Sources
Calcium	• Milk • Yogurt • Fortified soymilk • Kale • Broccoli • Spinach
Phosphorous (too much is actually detrimental to bone health)	• Protein-containing foods • Processed foods • Beverages that contain phosphoric acid
Vitamin D (it is difficult to obtain adequate dietary vitamin D; therefore, for individuals who live at high latitudes or spend little time outdoors, supplementation is recommended)	• Salmon • Fortified cereals • Milk (fortified) • Sunshine!
Magnesium	• Nuts and seeds • Halibut • Spinach • Beans
Vitamin K	• Turnip greens • Brussels sprouts • Broccoli • Spinach • Green leaf lettuce
Fluoride (children who drink water without fluoride should be prescribed a supplement by their doctor or dentist)	• Generally found in municipal drinking water

for good bone health and inadequate protein consumption can result in poor bone mineralization.

Key Points

Micronutrients serve many essential functions in the body ; for example, the B vitamins are required for the metabolism of carbohydrates, proteins and fats; vitamins A, C, and E act as antioxidants; and iron is essential for red blood cell production. Athletes can meet their micronutrients needs from a varied diet that includes an adequate intake of fruits, vegetables, whole grains, and dairy food (including dairy alternatives) and typically do not require a multivitamin supplement.

Hydration

Proper hydration practices are among the most important and easiest things an athlete can do to perform to potential. Adequate hydration before and during exercise enhances blood flow to the working muscles and improves thermoregulation. After exercise, fluid replacement is required for the effective transport of nutrients to the cells as well as decreasing heart rate and blood pressure back to normal resting homeostatic values.

Dehydration occurs when water losses are greater than water consumption. Exercise, heat, altitude, fever, vomiting, and diarrhea can dramatically increase fluid and, in some cases, electrolyte losses; if these losses are not quickly replaced, dehydration can rapidly result. Initiating a training session in a dehydrated state or allowing oneself to become dehydrated during a training session impairs performance and reduces the body's ability to regulate body temperature. As a result, dehydrated athletes are much more likely to suffer heat exhaustion and heat stroke compared to those who are properly hydrated.

Prolonged, high-intensity exercise in a warm environment is a common cause of dehydration because, in an effort to cool the body via evaporation, sweat rate can exceed 40 to 60 ounces per hour (1.2 to 1.8 L per hour); that is about 3 to 4 pounds or 1 to 2 kg of body weight each hour. Some fluid loss during exercise is to be expected and losing less than 2 percent of normal (euhydrated) body weight over the course of a training session is not dangerous and will not impair performance. Fluid losses greater than 2 percent of total euhydrated body weight may impair endurance performance because dehydration causes a reduction in sweat rate which impedes the body's ability to dissipate heat and results in an increase in core body temperature. When this occurs, perceived exertion and fatigue increases and if core body temperature becomes too high, heat exhaustion or heat stroke will occur.

Hydration Guidelines

Fluid needs vary greatly between and within individuals. Duration and intensity of physical activity, environmental conditions, and personal sweat rate are the greatest determinants of fluid needs. In general, urine should be light in color, almost like lemonade; it should never be dark yellow or brown, and a well-hydrated athlete should need to urinate every 90 minutes or so. General guidelines developed by the American College of Sports Medicine and in association with the National Athletic Trainers Association and the Academy for Nutrition and Dietetics can be found in Table 1.10.

Those exercising in extreme environments such as heat, cold, high and low humidity, or high altitude may have additional fluid needs by as much as 32 to 64 ounces each day. During seasonal weather changes or when traveling to new environments it is important to pay attention to these increased fluid needs.

What to Drink

Water is the best beverage choice for hydrating throughout the day. It contains no calories, has no sugar, nothing artificial, and no additives. Sweat is made up of water and electrolytes such as sodium therefore, if an athlete is sweating heavily, these electrolytes need to be replaced. Sports drinks are good sources of easily digested carbohydrates, electrolytes (sodium), and fluids. Under certain conditions, (such as existing low glycogen stores, continuous exercise >90

Table 1.10 General hydration guidelines for before, during, and after exercise

Activity	1 Hour before	During	After (Consume Slowly over the Course of an Hour)
Endurance sports	14–16 oz	5–12 oz every 15–20 minutes	24 oz for every pound lost during exercise
Team/winter sports	14–20 oz	4–5 oz every 10–15 minutes	24 oz for every pound lost during exercise

minutes, intermittent exercise >120 minutes, multiple training sessions a day, and/or lower than recommended daily carbohydrate or kcal intake) consuming sport drink may enhance performance when consumed prior to, during, or immediately after exercise. Because these products generally contain a 5- to 8-percent solution of glucose and fructose and a little added sodium, they are less likely to cause stomach upset or cramping compared to more highly concentrated fruit juice, energy drinks, soda, or candies. Sports drink contains about 60 kcal per 8 oz serving, or about 15 g of carbohydrate, and 150 to 200 mg of sodium. Energy drinks contain much more sugar and often have caffeine which increases risk of stomach upset and slows the absorption of fluids and carbohydrates. These products will also be discussed in Chapter 5.

Hyponatremia

Hyponatremia technically means low blood sodium and occurs as a result of ingesting large volumes of water in a short period of time. Excessive fluid, especially water, intake causes a decrease in the amount of sodium in the blood and can be very dangerous, even fatal. To prevent hyponatremia, it is important to drink fluids with electrolytes (sodium and potassium) and avoid drinking too much water or only water during long-duration exercise. Weight loss due to fluid loss during exercise is normal and not dangerous as long as those losses are minimized during exercise and replaced after exercise. Gaining weight from overdrinking is more dangerous than not drinking enough.

Key Points

Adequate body fluids are required to distribute oxygen and other nutrients to working muscle cells; body fluids are also needed to prevent dangerous exercise-induced increases in core body temperature. Therefore, appropriate hydration practices are an essential component of an effective sports nutrition plan. Water should be used to hydrate throughout the day and sport drink can be used during long-duration exercise or exercise in the heat. Post-exercise, about 24 ounces of fluid should be consumed for each pound of body weight lost. Avoid over-consumption of fluids as this is more dangerous than under-drinking.

Conclusion

Overall athletes can ensure they are meeting their macro- and micronutrient needs by consuming a balanced and varied diet. A whole foods-based diet that includes plentiful servings of fruits, vegetables, whole grains, lean protein sources, and dairy will provide athletes with a solid nutrition foundation that supports optimal training, recovery, and performance. Proper nutrition habits will improve an athlete's resiliency to infection and injury and allow for intense training and adaptation. Athletes should not separate their health from their performance, and nutrition habits bring these two components together.

All athletes should have a basic understanding of how the food they consume provides the fuel for their sport and should appreciate the relationship between health and performance. This chapter has established the foundation of sports nutrition principles; the following chapters will provide guidance and recommendations on how to implement these guidelines and problem-solve common challenges and issues that may arise.

References and Additional Readings

Thomas DT, et al. 2016. Position of the Academy of Nutrition and Dietetics, Dietitians of Canada, and the American College of Sports Medicine: Nutrition and Athletic Performance. *J Acad Nutr Diet.* 116, pp. 501–528.

American College of Sports Medicine, et al. 2007. American College of Sports Medicine Position Stand. Exercise and fluid replacement. *Med Sci Sports Exerc.* 39, no. 2, pp. 377–390.

Dunford M and Doyle JA. 2015. *Nutrition for Sport and Exercise, 3rd edition.* Stamford, CT. Cengage Learning Publishing.

Larson A. 2016. *Fuel for Sport: The Basics, 1st edition.* New York, NY. Momentum Press, LLC.

McArdle WD, et al. 2015. *Exercise Physiology: Nutrition, Energy, and Human Performance, 8th edition.* Baltimore, MD. Lippincott, Williams & Wilkins.

Academy of Nutrition and Dietetics. *Sports, Cardiovascular, and Wellness Nutrition.* http://www.scandpg.org/

Woodruff K. 2016. *Sports Nutrition.* New York, NY. Momentum Press, LLC.

CHAPTER 2

Optimal Eating for Optimal Training

Introduction

Much of the nutrition information in medical journals, textbooks, and popular media sources can seem abstract, even contradictory, as well as exceedingly difficult to put into practice. Science has a way of overcomplicating basic nutrition tenants, and media has a way of sensationalizing the latest research findings. The telephone game between science and the media, and the media to the consumer, generally results in a mistaken message that misses the larger context. Eating well and eating with the intent of *balance* is not, and should not, be overly complicated. Humans have been eating for thousands of years and, when highly processed foods stay out of the mix, we do a pretty good job fulfilling our nutrient requirements.

This chapter is intended to help the reader simplify and distill nutrition information and put recommendations into practice with simple strategies to overcome real-life barriers to eating nutritious foods at home, school, work, and when traveling to and from competitions. Specific recommendations regarding what and how much to eat before, during, and after exercise is also addressed using real-world scenarios and sport-specific nutrition guidance.

Develop a Food and Hydration Strategy for Optimal Performance

Athletes must support daily training with wise nutrition and hydration choices throughout the day, *every day*. Athletes spend a great deal of time training for optimal performance and those efforts should be supported with nutrient-dense, unprocessed foods in the correct amounts and at the appropriate times.

Many athletes want to know what to eat the night or morning before a big event. While the pregame meal is important, consistent optimal performance is best achieved through diligent training, proper recovery practices, and daily attention to personal nutrition and hydration demands. In order to train optimally, one must eat optimally; therefore, it is necessary to consider and plan what, how much, and when food will be eaten *each day—not just race day.*

Planning ahead and having a food and hydration strategy can help an athlete navigate otherwise-difficult nutrition choices and scenarios that often result in poor choices or skipping meals. A food and hydration strategy also fosters healthy eating habits and allows the athlete to prepare and fuel in such a way as to promote optimal training, recovery, and overall health. These habits can also help ensure adequate macro- and micronutrient intake, minimize digestive problems, and can serve as a source of predictable comfort.

The first step to putting together a food and hydration strategy for optimal training and recovery is to determine what and when foods are already being eaten. Haphazard eating is common among Americans, especially teens, and can lead to poor overall eating patterns. This style of unplanned eating can lead to the consumption of too many calories and too few nutrients but can also lead to inadequate carbohydrate, protein, and fluid intake at times that are critical for optimal training and recovery. Meals and snacks are often skipped among high school and college athletes but going without food for a prolonged period of time (>3 to 4 hours) may result in low blood sugar levels which can decrease mental and physical acuity. Most athletes who train daily need three meals and two to three snacks to maintain optimal physical and mental performance. Breakfast is probably the meal most commonly skipped among all populations, and on any given day up to 20 percent of school-age children and 31 percent of adolescents skip breakfast.

In order to better understand current dietary patterns and subsequently improve overall nutrition, one can complete a 3-day food record or a 24-hour food recall. All dietary assessments should be completed as honestly and precisely as possible and include specifics such as time and amount of foods and fluids consumed. Forms should also reflect usual dietary patterns with as few deviations from the typical diet as possible. If access to a nutrition professional is available, this person can analyze diet records and give recommendations regarding daily eating habits. Less accurate but more convenient are online nutrient assessment tools.

Estimating energy, carbohydrate, protein, fat, and fluid needs is the second step to developing a comprehensive food and hydration strategy. Assessment of current intake means little without estimated values of what, how much, and when foods and fluids should be consumed. These details depend on training demands, current body weight and composition, and body weight/composition goals. Chapter 1 provides detailed information and examples for the estimation of energy, macronutrient, and fluid needs.

The third step to developing a food and hydration strategy involves comparing dietary intake with dietary needs. In general, dietary goals should include meeting one's predetermined calorie, macronutrient (protein, carbohydrates, and fat), and micronutrient (vitamins and minerals) needs (see Chapter 1 to calculate estimated macronutrient needs). Optimal eating also includes the consumption of whole grains (rather than refined grains), whole fruits (rather than juice), vegetables (not just potatoes or corn!), lean sources of protein, and dairy (unless lactose intolerant or allergic to milk). Unfortunately a lot of athletes consume sugary breakfast cereals and breakfast bars, pastries, chips, refined white bread, French fries, fast-food hamburgers, fruit-*flavored* beverages, and fruit snacks that have no fruit. These highly processed foods provide little in the way of nutrients and likely increase the inflammation process in the body. These foods also have long-term consequences in regard to eventual insulin resistance, overweight/obesity, and increased risk for chronic disease. A food and hydration strategy can help reduce intake of these highly processed foods as can an understanding of the most recent updates to the USDA Dietary Recommendations: https://health.gov/dietaryguidelines/2015/guidelines/

Once usual intake has been assessed and results compared to estimated needs, specific strengths and weaknesses should be identified and, from this information, goals can be developed. An individual food and hydration strategy should aim to meet an athlete's estimated carbohydrate, protein, fat, and fluid needs and improve on dietary shortcomings. Rather than revamping an entire way of eating, the food and hydration strategy should build off of existing strengths and normal dietary patterns but should be continuously revised and tweaked to meet changing food and fluid needs. The food and hydration strategy is also very useful for identifying optimal *time* for food and fluid consumption; many athletes meet personal fluid, macronutrient, and micronutrient needs but would be better able to utilize those nutrients if consumed at different times. A food and hydration strategy can make an athlete more likely to consume nutrients exactly when they are needed most.

Food and Hydration Strategies for Breakfast

For many children and adults, breakfast is an afterthought (if even a thought at all). Along with not being hungry, lack of time is one of the most commonly cited reasons children do not eat breakfast. It is easy to overlook breakfast during the morning hustle and bustle. Mornings often involve a constant state of rushing to and from practice, class, work, or trying to get a few extra minutes of sleep. In the midst of all the juggling, good eating habits are often neglected. However, with some simple strategies and planning, it is possible to make time for nutritious and convenient breakfast options.

Breakfast is important even putting athletics aside. There is much research-based evidence to suggest that skipping breakfast causes a decrease in academic performance. Students who eat breakfast score better on tests, have an overall higher GPA, miss less school, and have better nutrition habits compared to non-breakfast eaters. Some of these findings may not necessarily be cause and effect but the results make physiological sense and eating breakfast certainly cannot *hurt* cognitive prowess.

Eating breakfast helps to maintain blood glucose levels throughout the morning. Failure to eat a morning meal may cause a midmorning drop in blood glucose, which decreases the ability to focus and concentrate. Low blood glucose also leads to feelings of intense hunger, and an overly hungry breakfast skipper is more likely to make poor food choices later in the day (i.e., the midmorning raid of the vending machine). When blood sugar crashes, nutritionally wise choices are not on the radar and often the quick fix is something high in sugar and low in protein and fiber. These highly processed foods cause a large spike in blood sugar which in turn causes a spike in insulin. When this happens, sugar from the blood rushes into the cells and within an hour or two there is very little glucose left in the circulating blood and leaves the central nervous system without adequate fuel, thus setting the stage for another crash. This early afternoon drop in blood glucose often occurs just prior to after-school sports practice and can leave an athlete dragging. Therefore, skipping breakfast not only hampers morning academic performance but also afternoon sport performance.

If an athlete trains in the morning, breakfast becomes even more important. Without good nutrition and hydration habits the recovery from morning training sessions is much slower and the risk of becoming dehydrated and/or glycogen depleted increases. All this leads to less energy for school and training later in the day.

Athletes make time for training and also should make time to fuel that training. To train, recover, compete, and even think optimally an athlete must eat optimally from start to finish every day. This requires planning and preparation. For example, each evening an athlete can prepare the next day's breakfast by packing a quick to-go bag with a piece of fruit, yogurt, granola or a peanut butter and jelly sandwich, so in the morning all that is required is opening up the fridge and grabbing the sack!

What is eaten for breakfast is also important. Common choices among teens and young adults include highly refined convenience foods such as donuts, sugared cereals, and packaged cookies and crackers. These choices lack protein and fiber and will cause the previously described insulin spike and subsequent rapid decrease in blood glucose.

A balanced breakfast supports an athlete's training demands and includes a source of carbohydrate, protein, fat, and fiber. For example, fresh fruit, whole wheat toast, two scrambled eggs, and possibly a glass of milk or cup of yogurt. Although a hard sell for teenagers, we can attempt to encourage athletes to wake up 20 or 30 minutes earlier to make time for such a breakfast but considering the audience it may be easier to herd cats. Of course there are other more convenient, yet still adequate, options. Peanut butter and jelly on whole wheat bread with a glass of milk; a bowl of raisin bran with low-fat milk and a banana; or yogurt topped with granola can all meet the athlete's nutrient needs. Table 2.1 provides ideas for a mix-and-match breakfast system that provides about 400 calories; if additional calories are needed just add another protein, carbohydrate, or fat choice.

Many athletes are not hungry in the morning; these individuals can try eating an hour or so after they get to school or work. For example, a yogurt smoothie, either made at home or bought from the grocery store and a half sandwich can be kept in an insulated lunch bag and stored in a locker or backpack. Sport bars are also convenient and not overly filling but not all are created equally. Many bars are just expensive, vitamin-fortified candy, made with unwholesome ingredients, such as high-fructose corn syrup and partially hydrogenated oils. A sport bar without a candy coating, which are usually the sources of hydrogenated oils and other questionable ingredients, and includes 3 to 4 g of fiber, 20 to 40 g of carbohydrate, and 8 to 12 g of protein, makes for a good choice. Brands

Table 2.1 Breakfast mix and match. Choose at least one item from each category for a 400- to 500-kcal balanced breakfast. If additional calories are needed, add another carbohydrate, fat, and/or protein

Carbohydrates (50 g)	Protein (10–15 g)	Fat (5–10 g)
1½ cup Wheaties or other whole-grain cereal and ½ cup sliced strawberries	8–12 oz low-fat milk or soy milk	1 oz almonds or other nuts
Two pieces toast and banana	One egg + egg whites	1 oz cheese or cream cheese
1 cup cooked oatmeal and ¼ cup dried fruit	8–12 oz soy milk or yogurt	1 tbsp peanut butter, almond butter, or sunflower butter
½ cup granola and 1 oz of raisins	2 oz "light" or reduced fat cheese or soy cheese	½ avocado or ¼ cup reduced-sugar or no-sugar-added coconut flakes
One large whole wheat tortilla or two small tortillas and ¼ cup salsa or chopped tomatoes	One egg and 1 oz cheese	2 tbsp light sour cream
One large whole wheat bagel	Two eggs	1 tbsp butter
1 cup whole oats (oatmeal)	One egg and ½ cup milk	1 oz sunflower seeds
Four graham crackers	12 oz low-fat chocolate milk	1 tbsp Nutella

such as Clifbar, Luna, Mojo, Lara, Power Bar Harvest, and Power Bar Nut Natural fall into this category, as do many others, but it is important to take a look at the nutrition facts and ingredient list because content and quality vary greatly among and even within brands.

Breakfast can also be split into two parts, individuals can have something small, such as a Greek yogurt before leaving in the morning, followed by a piece of fruit and a sports bar a couple hours later. Eating two mini-meals can seem less offensive to the athlete who claims to have no appetite in the morning.

In an ideal world everyone would have time to sit down and eat a relaxed, wholesome breakfast such as a spinach omelet with whole-wheat toast, or oatmeal topped with fresh fruit and yogurt. But breakfast can also be a quick, convenient, leftovers from last night's dinner taken in a Tupperware, eaten on the go. There is no need to limit the first meal of the day to traditional breakfast foods. The point is to start the day with healthy foods in order to feel and perform well for the rest of the day. For more breakfast recipes, refer to Chapter 6.

Key Points

Breakfast is essential for success in sport and school. Planning and sourcing food for breakfast is very important, especially for athletes who have morning and afternoon training sessions. Breakfast options do not have to be elaborate but should be healthy and include a balanced proportion of carbohydrates, proteins, and fats.

Food and Hydration Strategies for Lunch

Lunch is no less important than breakfast, especially considering it is generally consumed just prior to or just after training. Athletes need healthy sources of carbohydrates, proteins, and fats for energy and building muscle. Athletes also need natural sources of vitamins, minerals, and phytonutrients for recovery and a strong immune system. Soda and greasy pizza that is finished off with an ice cream sandwich is not an athlete's lunch.

Brown bagging is the best option but does take time and planning; however, in return, this strategy can allow for an athlete to consume preplanned, quantified, nutritious, and balanced fuel and fluids at the most appropriate time. Familiar foods and appropriately timed eating can also minimize risk of gastrointestinal (GI) upset later in the day as well as ensure that an athlete is getting what is wanted and needed. Why overpay for mediocre cafeteria food or fast food with questionable ingredients and nutritional value?

A well-balanced lunch can take on many appearances and does not have to be the standard, sometimes monotonous, sandwich on whole wheat, apple, baby carrots, and milk. There are dozens of convenient lunch variations that can be conveniently packed into lidded plastic to-go containers, many of which are leftovers from the night before!

Balanced lunch 500 to 800 kcal ideas (pair with 8-oz low-fat milk and 8-oz water)**:

- Two to three slices of homemade pizza with a piece of fruit
- 2 cups meat or tofu stir-fry with vegetables and 1 cup of brown rice
- One or two pieces of "athlete lasagna" (recipe located in Chapter 6) and one piece of fruit
- 2 cups of a bean, rice, cheese, and salsa combination (diced peppers and tomatoes are also a tasty addition)
- Two large whole grain pancakes with diced fruit and 6 oz of Greek yogurt
- 2 to 3 cups of "super salads" topped with 2 oz of a protein source and a 2-oz chunk of whole-grain bread
- 1 to 2 cups of pasta or potato salad made with low-fat dressing, diced chicken, and veggies
- 1 to 2 cups of "power" macaroni and cheese made with spinach and tomatoes and a piece of fruit
- 1 cup fruit, 1 cup Greek yogurt, and ½ cup granola for a delicious parfait (additional granola and/or nuts can be added for those with larger appetites)
- Homemade Lunchable with 2 oz whole grain crackers, 1 oz cheese and/or 1 oz lunch meat, one serving of fruit, 1 cup sugar snap peas (or other favorite vegetable), and ½ cup trail mix

- Multigrain waffle sandwich with nut butter, jelly, and a banana (most athletes will need two of these)
- 1 to 2 cups of soup in a thermos and a big chunk (2 to 3 oz) of whole grain bread, 1 to 2 oz cheese, and a piece of fruit

*Lunch items such as meat, eggs, and dairy should be kept cold in an insulated lunch bag containing an ice pack; if desired food can be reheated just prior to eating.

While packing lunch is preferable to purchasing a cafeteria-sourced lunch, in some circumstances this is unavoidable. In these cases athletes should aim for a meal that includes the following four components: a whole grain source, a lean protein, fruits and vegetables, and a dairy (or dairy alternative) option. Sometimes there is a featured *healthy choice* entrée served in the cafeteria that provides these foods, such as a black bean burrito on a whole wheat tortilla, a piece of fruit and side salad, and a glass of milk. Other cafeterias may have a la carte options. Good choices in this arena include veggie burgers and grilled chicken burgers on some type of whole-grain bread. Ideally this is paired with a glass of milk and a piece of fruit as well as a salad created from the salad bar with mixed greens and vegetables, possibly topped with nuts and seeds. Avoiding fried and other foods high in fat pays big dividends later in the day (and life!), as these foods often increase risk of GI distress while training and offer little in terms of health and performance benefits. Other common choices such as chips, sugary baked goods, sugared beverages, and candy should also be reconsidered and replaced with more wholesome choices such as plain milk, whole fruits, nuts, and string cheese, as these selections will positively improve performance, recovery, and overall health. Creating awareness among athletes regarding healthy choices will help to influence positive food choices.

Food and Hydration Strategies for Training and Competition

How soon and what to eat before a training session or competition is a common query. In reality there is no *magic meal* but NOT eating OR eating the *wrong* foods can hinder performance. Too little food or fluids and the body would not have nutrients needed for thinking, competing, and recovering. The wrong kinds of food or too much food may leave an athlete feeling sluggish or even sick due to GI distress. In the case of too much food, performance can be hampered because large meals cause blood to go to the gut in an effort to digest instead of going to working muscles. Food intake prior to training and competition is a balancing act of not too much but not too little. The following information should help to clarify some of the pretraining/competition nutrition enigmas.

Pretraining and Competition Meals

In general, meals should be eaten at least 2 to 3 hours before training/competing. A good pretraining/precompetition meal should be high in carbohydrate, moderate in protein, and low in fat. High-protein, high-fat, and high-fiber foods stay in the stomach longer, are more difficult to digest and, in some individuals, may cause stomach upset. Since each person has his or her unique tolerances, an athlete's best precompetition meal should be determined via trial and error in the off-season or pre-season. The day before and day of a competition should always include familiar foods, as this is never the time to experiment with a precompetition meal! Even the seemingly healthy whole wheat pancakes served at the race may appear to be a good idea, but if the athlete has never consumed these before, they may find themselves making unnecessary (and performance-hindering) trips to the bathroom! For some athletes this means that, when on the road, they pack personal precompetition meals to ensure they have access to familiar foods.

A good precompetition morning meal eaten 3 hours before the event may look like this:

- 1 cup of Wheaties
- ¾ cup 1 percent milk
- One banana
- One piece of toast with 1 tbsp peanut butter
- 12 oz water

This meal will provide about 16 g of protein, 15 g of fat, and 100 g of carbohydrates and about 500 to 600 kcals.

Regularly consumed and easily digestible foods are the best option prior to competition. It is also important to be well hydrated; good choices include water, diluted juice, or sports drink. Consuming a small snack or some sports drink 30 to 60 minutes before training or competition can also be beneficial. If a snack is eaten make sure it is something that is low in protein and fat, such as a banana, so that it can be used for quick energy.

Strategies for Recovery Nutrition

Proper recovery nutrition is important for all athletes. After an intense workout or competition it is important to refuel the body. Muscles need carbohydrates to replace glycogen and protein to repair and hypertrophy muscles. Recovery nutrition includes carbohydrates, proteins, fats with omega-3s, electrolytes (sodium, potassium, and magnesium), and fluids. Fluids are especially important. After practice or competition it is recommended to drink about 20 to 24 oz, or about one large Gatorade bottle, of fluid per pound of sweat-induced losses in body weight. This should not be consumed all at once but rather spread out over a period of a few hours. An athlete can weigh themselves before and after practice to calculate lost water weight. Sweat also contains salt and athletes should replace these losses via sodium-containing beverages, such as Gatorade. Normal sodium losses can be replaced through standard dietary intake but sports drink can be helpful during periods of heat acclimation or excessive sweating. *Salty sweaters* may also benefit from additional sodium intake. A salty sweater can be identified by the crusty white salt on exercise clothing or on one's skin.

After training or competition a mixture of carbohydrate and protein should be consumed within 30 to 60 minutes to start the process of replacing glycogen and to help repair damaged muscles. Rehydration during this postexercise window is also important and can be enhanced by consuming electrolyte-containing fluids. Many athletes may not feel like eating solid food immediately following a workout; in these instances drinking a beverage such as chocolate milk will deliver all of the essentials: fluids, electrolytes, carbohydrates, and protein.

When choosing recovery foods aim for the following:
- 50 g of carbohydrate
- 10 g of protein
- 24 oz of fluids
- Within 60 minutes of hard training

Recovery foods include the following:
- Low-fat milk with cereal
- Sport bars (Powerbar, Clifbar, etc.)
- Low-fat chocolate milk
- Turkey or ham and cheese sandwich
- Yogurt
- Fruit smoothie made with milk or yogurt

Eating as soon as possible after an intense workout or competition is essential for quick recovery and will help to prepare the body for the next training session. It is especially important to eat after training when an athlete has two-a-day workouts, is at a training camp, or when they have back-to-back matches and need to recover quickly.

Sports drinks, chocolate milk, and energy bars are great options for initiating the recovery process but an athlete should also plan on having a well-balanced meal within 2 hours postexercise to complete the nutrition recovery process. Preparing for post-training and post-competition nutrient needs is essential for optimal recovery and health. Information related to nutrition and hydration needs before, during, and after training is summarized in Table 2.2.

Postcompetition meals ideas:
- Pasta with chicken and vegetables
- Stir-fry with rice
- Turkey burger on a big multigrain bun
- Multigrain pancakes with fruit
- Burrito with chicken and beans (easy on the cheese)
- Turkey and avocado sandwich with a bowl of fruit

Table 2.2 *Approximate timing and intake guidelines before, during, and after intense training and competition*

Situation	Fluid Goals	Carbohydrate Goals	Protein Goals	Food Examples
2–4 Hours before Training or Competition	16 oz of water	1–4 g/kg or 50–400 g (depends on time prior to activity and individual tolerance)	15–20 g	• 1 cup milk + 2 cups cereal + one banana OR • One bagel + 2 tbsp peanut butter + one apple + 10 oz milk OR • One to two poached eggs + two pieces toast + one orange + 10 oz milk OR • 2 cups of pasta with tomato sauce + ½ cup diced chicken
30–60 min. before Training or Competition	8–16 oz water (depends on sweat rate and climate)	30–50 g	Up to 10 g PRO may be beneficial	• One sport bar* (8–10 g PRO) + 8 oz sport drink • ½ cup Greek yogurt with ¼ cup granola • Half to one bagel w/1 tbsp light cream cheese • 5–10 crackers + 1 oz cheese
During Training or Competition >60–90 minutes	20–32 oz sport drink or water	1 g/minute or 30–60 g per hour	Small amounts of BCAA possibly beneficial	Sport gel or other CHO supplement if sport drink is not consumed
Recovery 30–60 min. post-training especially important for two-a-day sessions or multiple-event days	16–32 oz fluid (depends on sweat rate)	1 g/kg or 50–70 g	10–15 g	• 2 cups sport drink + sport bar • 2 cups sport drink + peanut butter or turkey sandwich • 12 oz low-fat chocolate milk • 1 cup fruit yogurt

* Sports bar with at least 8–10 g of protein

** 1 cup of yogurt with about 8–10 g of protein

Food and Hydration Strategies for Snacks and Eating on the Road

Young athletes spend a lot of time at school, practice, and traveling to and from competitive events. Eating away from home can result in poor nutritional choices, and it can be a challenge to keep a regular eating pattern and choose healthy foods. At the school cafeteria, during travel, and when out with friends, it is crucial to make good nutrition choices each day and not just the night before or morning of a competitive event.

Plan ahead! Athletes should take a few extra minutes before leaving for school, a road trip, or heading out for training/competition to make sure foods that will fuel their performance and recovery are available. It is important athletes learn early on that it is their responsibility to fuel themselves well and do not fall into the habit of *haphazard eating*. This is the kind of eating where the nutritional quality of the food is not considered and they end up eating whatever is available, is convenient, or looks appetizing. Even packing peanut butter, jelly, bread, and some fresh fruit can make all the difference between having a nutritious, familiar meal before a competition and having no alternative except fried food from a fast food restaurant, or a bag of chips from a vending machine.

A good first step to avoiding haphazard eating is to teach athletes how to create a food *travel pack*. These can be used for snacks at school, work, before practice, after practice, and on the road. Travel packs are especially helpful in the event there is limited time to stop for food on the way to or from an event, if restaurant selections are limited or do not have many nutritious selections, or if athletes are going to be in any sort of situation where food convenience and options are unknown. Travel packs are also great options for athletes who have before and after school practices.

Travel pack items that neatly fit into a sports bag and can be toted along on trips include the following (C = good source of carbohydrates, P = good source of protein, F = food has a high fat content):

- Dried fruit (C)
- Beef or turkey jerky (P)
- Low-fat chocolate or strawberry milk (C, P)
- Nuts (P, F)
- Nature Valley or Kashi granola bars (C)

- Pretzels (C)
- Animal crackers (C)
- Whole fruits, apples/bananas/oranges (C)
- Vegetables, baby carrots, cherry tomatoes, cucumber slices, celery sticks
- Bagels (C)
- Sports bars, Cliff bars, Luna bars, Powerbar Harvest (C, P)
- Sandwiches (C, P, F depending on the type)
- Dry ready-to-eat cereal (C)
- Fruit yogurt (C, P)
- Water!
- Sports drinks (C)

Remember to rinse fruits and veggies before packing them in a baggie and keep perishable foods (fresh fruit and vegetables, deli meat, and dairy products) in a cooler with ice or a freezer pack during travel. Many of the above food items also make for nutritiously sound snacks (avoid sports drink except for training purposes).

Eating Out

Packing healthy meals when traveling is ideal. However, when this is not possible, restaurant fair does not have to be burgers and fries. Nutritious choices can be found most anywhere including fast food venues. In general athletes can look for menu options that include a whole grain/starch, a lean protein, and fruits and/or vegetables. Athletes should be nutrition conscious when eating out; the following tips may help:

- Restaurant portions are generally very oversized; don't feel obligated to "clean your plate".
- Choose a large salad as the main meal with the dressing on the side.
- Choose whole grains like whole wheat bread and pasta, brown rice, and oatmeal when available.

- Order fruit, soup, or salad on the side instead of French fries, coleslaw, or mashed potatoes and gravy.
- Request to have salad dressing on the side and use sparingly.
- If ordering pizza, select thin crust (whole grain if available) with veggies instead of sausage or pepperoni.
- Order sandwiches without sauces or mayonnaise or choose mustard.
- Ask for an extra side order of fruit or vegetables.
- Order pasta dishes that are made with marinara sauce and easy on the cheese.
- Choose skim or low-fat milk and yogurts.
- Avoid cream sauces.
- Avoid fried or breaded starches and vegetables.
- Choose lean meat that have been broiled or grilled, avoid deep-fried or breaded meats.
- Stay well hydrated—athletes should carry a water bottle and use it! They should be encouraged to avoid soda, energy, and juice drinks.

Key Points

Athletes should be encouraged to focus on healthy, nutritious meals and snacks, not just when at home but at school, on the road, and when eating out. Simple strategies that include choosing whole grains and starches, fruits and vegetables, and lean proteins can be used to select balanced meals that will meet the athlete's nutrient and energy needs. Athletes need to be aware of the importance of timing nutrient intake appropriately. Consuming adequate carbohydrate and fluids prior to exercise and immediately post-exercise is especially important for performance and recovery. Overall being prepared and planning ahead will save time and ultimately support optimal performance.

References and Additional Readings

Ament W and Verkerke GJ. 2009. Exercise and fatigue. *Sports Med.* 39, no. 5, pp. 389–422.

American College of Sports Medicine, et al. 2007. American College of Sports Medicine Position Stand. Exercise and fluid replacement. *Med Sci Sports Exerc.* 39, no. 2, pp. 377–390.

Baker LB, et al. 2015. Acute effects of carbohydrate supplementation on intermittent sport performance. *Nutrients.* 7, pp. 5733–5763.

Beaven CM, et al. 2013. Effects of caffeine and carbohydrate mouth rinses on repeated sprint performance. *Appl Physiol Nutr Metab.* 38, no. 6, pp. 633–637.

Cermak NM and van Loon LJ. 2013. The use of carbohydrates during exercise as an ergogenic aid. *Sports Med.* 43, no. 11, pp. 1139–1155.

D'anci KE, et al. 2009. Voluntary dehydration and cognitive performance in trained college athletes. *Percept Mot Skills.* 109, no. 1, pp. 251–269.

Larson A. 2016. *Fuel for Sport: The Basics, 1ˢᵗ edition.* New York, NY. Momentum Press, LLC.

USDA Dietary Recommendations. *Dietary Guidelines for Americans 2015–2020.* https://health.gov/dietaryguidelines/2015/guidelines/.

CHAPTER 3

Energy Balance, Body Weight, and Body Composition

Introduction to Energy Balance

Energy balance refers to the amount of energy (kcals) eaten relative to the amount of energy expended. A positive energy balance refers to the state when more kcals are eaten than expended. A positive energy balance is necessary for growth, increasing muscle mass, and weight gain. Athletes who are still growing should generally be in a positive energy balance. A negative energy balance refers to the state when fewer kcals are eaten than expended. A negative energy balance will facilitate the breakdown of fat stores and possibly muscle in order to meet daily energy demands. An equal energy balance refers to the state when energy intake is the same as the energy required for resting metabolic rate, the thermic effect of food, and physical activity. An equal energy balance is required to maintain a given body weight within a few pounds; normal daily fluctuations in weight typically represent changes in hydration status as fat or muscle mass will not change significantly on a day-to-day basis.

The balancing act of equalizing energy in to energy out usually happens over a period of several days or even weeks, but ultimately an equal energy balance provides a sufficient number of calories to train, compete, and maintain an optimal weight. In order to maintain this balance there are times when an athlete may need to consume more energy (kcals), as is the case when training volume and/or exercise intensity increases. There are also times when an athlete will require fewer calories to maintain this balance, for example, during training tapers, the off-season, during times of injury, or any other reason which causes a decrease in training volume and/or intensity. In the event an athlete continues to eat the same amount of food in either scenario there may be unwanted weight losses or gains, respectively.

Specific energy needs depend on several factors:
- Frequency, duration, and intensity of training
- Physical activity outside of training
- Current body weight and body composition
- Goal body weight
- Rate of growth
- Genetic factors

Energy requirements for athletes vary greatly and can range from 2,300 to 4,500 calories per day, but it is not necessary to count calories in or calories out to maintain, gain, or even lose body weight. If an athlete wants to know how many calories he or she should be consuming on a daily basis, a sports dietitian can assess daily energy needs by conducting an in-depth assessment of his or her body weight, body composition, training demands, and other daily activities. But as a general rule of thumb, an athlete who maintains his or her weight over time is likely consuming adequate calories for weight maintenance. An exception to this includes athletes who chronically restrict daily intake and consequently blunt resting metabolic rate. If an athlete's weight is increasing over time then energy intake is greater than total energy demands; if body weight is decreasing over time then too little energy is consumed relative to energy expenditure. However, a change in body weight does not indicate whether the weight gain or weight loss is in the form of lean body mass or fat mass; only body composition assessment can provide this information.

Key Points

Energy balance is achieved when as many calories are expended as consumed and weight remains stable. Positive and negative energy balances will cause weight gain and weight loss, respectively.

Weight Loss in Athletes

All athletes seek a competitive advantage, and some believe this edge can be attained via weight loss. Athletes in sports such as running, cycling, and rock climbing require a high strength-to-body-weight ratio and many believe that reductions in body weight will improve performance. Other sports include an aesthetic component, as is the case in gymnastics, figure skating, and diving. Judging the aesthetics of how an athlete appears can drive these competitors to seek a lower body weight in the hopes that it will improve overall scores. Athletes who compete in sports with specific weight classes may also believe that competing in lower weight classes offers a performance advantage. Finally some athletes believe the lighter they are the better they will perform regardless of sport.

Athletes should be educated that lighter is not always better and a lower body weight does not guarantee improved performance. All athletes have limitations on how much he or she can manipulate body weight. Genetic factors, frame size, and stage of pubertal development are not within an athlete's control. There is no *ideal* weight or percent of body fat for athletes competing in any given sport. Rather, athletes within a given sport will represent a *range* of a healthy weights and body compositions that support optimal performance. Athletes should be encouraged to compete at a weight that is appropriate for their age, height, frame size, and stage of growth and development (American Academy of Pediatrics Committee on Sports and Fitness 2005). This said, mature, elite athletes within a given sport will likely fall into a more narrow range of body weights and compositions.

If weight loss is deemed appropriate, the importance of supporting safe weight loss practices cannot be overemphasized. Chronic dieting and severe caloric restriction, as well as other unhealthy weight loss practices, can ultimately progress to the development of a diagnosed eating disorder. Athletes who choose to lose weight should not do so because of pressure from coaches, team members, or family members and should ideally work with a sports dietitian. More information regarding disordered eating and eating disorders among athletes can be found in Chapter 4.

Athletes who are overweight may see performance and health benefits from healthy weight loss; individuals already at a healthy weight are less likely to see performance benefits. In addition to body weight, *body composition*, the ratio of fat mass to fat-free mass expressed as percent body fat, must also be taken into consideration. This measurement is a better determinant as to whether weight loss is appropriate. Body Mass Index, or BMI, can be used to assess weight status but is simply a ratio of height to weight and does not specifically measure body composition. Athletes with increased muscle mass may have a higher BMI value, even though they may be quite lean. Assessment of body composition is a much more accurate way to determine if an athlete should lose weight. For example, if an athlete is seeking to lose 10 pounds but his or her percent body fat is already quite low, it would be advisable that this athlete reconsider his or her goal weight.

There are no body fat percentage minimums or maximums universally accepted as being *too low* or *too high*; however, in 2006 the National Federation of State High School Associations did adopt standards for body composition for wrestling. The standards require a body fat minimum of ≥7 percent for males and ≥12 percent for females. These minimums are higher than those established by the National Collegiate Athletic Association (NCAA), and this is to account for growth needs in adolescents (Turocy et al 2011). Furthermore, the Australian Institute of Sport recommends athletes who participate in sports with designated weights classes, compete in a class that is within 5 percent of their *current* body mass. This is to ensure excessive weight is not lost and weight that is lost is more likely to be maintained. Both standards can be applied to athletes of all sports.

Extreme weight loss practices include severely restricting calories, self-induced vomiting, excessive exercise, diet pill consumption, and voluntary dehydration using methods such as fluid restriction, diuretics/laxatives, excessive spitting, and use of saunas/rubber suits. All of these practices are strongly discouraged, are dangerous and have resulted in long-term eating disorders, hospitalizations, and even death.

The preferred approach to weight management, especially for younger athletes, is to place an emphasis on healthy eating, good training habits, and tracking changes in body composition. These practices help to ensure optimal training conditions for the athlete now and into the future and support overall health. Safe weight loss practices specifically include adequate intake of fluids, energy, and micronutrients in conjunction with a small to moderate calorie deficit and modest increases in exercise duration and frequency. A sports dietitian can provide nutrition recommendations and guidance on how to achieve individual weight loss goals.

Key Points

Many athletes feel pressures to attain a low body weight or ultra-lean body composition. Athletes should be educated that lighter is not always better and successful athletes come in all shapes and sizes. Athletes who wish to lose weight should have BMI and body composition assessed to determine realistic goals and ideally referred to a sport dietitian.

Weight Loss Strategies

Ideally body weight and body composition concerns among athletes are assessed and monitored by a sports dietitian. In general, coaches and trainers should refrain from making comments about an athlete's weight and avoid becoming overly involved in nutritional strategies intended to alter body size. This said, athletes often look to coaches and athletic trainers for dietary advice and sometimes advice as to how to gain or lose weight. In the event a dietitian is not accessible, the following information gives coaches, trainers, and other exercise professionals a briefing on safe weight loss.

If determined to be appropriate and potentially beneficial, weight loss should be gradual at a rate of 1 to 2 pounds per week. Weight loss at a more rapid rate (>2 pounds a week) can result in loss of muscle mass and is likely detrimental to performance. Appropriate weight loss should be addressed in the off-season or preseason; weight loss during competition season can impair performance due to compromised energy intake. During the weight loss period, body weight measurements should be taken at regular intervals about one to two times per week. Weights should be taken with minimal clothing and at the same time of day relative to exercise training and consumption of meals. Body weight should be assessed in private; group weigh-ins are strongly discouraged because this practice promotes negative body image issues. Body composition should also be assessed every 6 weeks and periodically throughout the year to gauge progress toward the athlete's goals and maintenance of these goals.

Once an appropriate amount of weight has been lost and the desired body composition is attained, both should be maintained and assessed periodically. Weight cycling, including frequent patterns of weight gain and weight loss, should be avoided as this can be detrimental to metabolic health and body composition. This is demonstrated by the fact that athletes who lose weight and maintain the new weight have higher resting metabolic rates than athletes who constantly weight cycle.

Weight loss requires creating an energy deficit via increased energy expenditure or a reduction in energy intake, or a combination of both. When energy intake is restricted, an individual may feel hungry, irritable, more easily fatigued, and risks nutrient deficiencies. Utilizing the concepts of nutrient and energy density can help to ameliorate these potential pitfalls. To review, energy in the foods we eat come from the macronutrients: carbohydrates, proteins, and fats. The amount of energy in a given amount of food can be quantified in terms of calories, or more commonly kcals. *Energy density* refers to the number of kcals per serving or in a given volume. Foods that are very high in calories are said to be *energy dense*. For example, cheese is quite energy dense and per 1 oz serving, a cube about the size of the average thumb, has approximately 100 kcals. An example of a food that is *not* energy dense is a cucumber, which has about 4 kcals per 1 oz, about half a cup diced. Choosing foods that have a low energy density allows an individual to eat a greater volume of food with fewer total kcals. This can be advantageous for someone who is trying to lose weight because, all other things being equal, a larger volume of food is more likely to satiate one's appetite compared to a smaller volume. Tables 3.1 and 3.2 list foods with high and low energy densities, respectively; foods listed in Table 3.2 also have a high nutrient density.

Energy density refers to caloric content but does not take into account *nutrient density*, which refers to vitamin, mineral, fiber, and phytonutrient content per serving or unit of volume. Many convenient and easily accessible energy dense foods have a low nutrient density. Most of the processed foods we turn to for meals and snacks have ample calories but are lacking in overall nutritional quality. On the other hand, many foods

Table 3.1 High energy density foods

Sugared beverages: soda, energy drinks, fruit-flavored drinks
Juice
Chocolate milk
Candies and chocolates
Pastries: donuts, muffins, croissants, cakes, pies, etc.
Cookies
Ice cream
Chips
Fried foods
Dried fruit
Liquid and solid fats: oils, butter, cream, mayonnaise, salad dressing
Nuts
Nut butters
Cheese and cream cheese

Table 3.2 Low energy density foods

All vegetables with the exception of corn and potatoes
All legumes (beans) with the exception of peanuts
All fresh and frozen fruit with the exception of coconuts and avocados
Low-fat dairy products without added sugar
Lean sources of protein such as fish, shrimp, egg whites, and chicken breast
Vinegars
Most noncream-based soups and broths

that are low in energy are very high in overall nutrients and are considered to be nutrient dense. Fruits and vegetables are excellent examples of foods with a low energy density but high nutrient density. For example, broccoli has only 30 kcals per cup but is loaded with vitamin C and is a good source of fiber and vitamin A; bananas have about 110 kcals per medium/large fruit and are an excellent source of potassium and fiber and a good source of vitamin C. Additionally, some energy dense foods are also very nutritious. Cheese is a good source of calcium and protein, and pistachios have healthy fats, fiber, and protein. Almonds, avocado, and most other nuts and seeds are other examples of nutrient and energy dense foods. Foods that are energy dense and nutrient dense can be part of a healthful diet even when trying to lose weight but portion size should be taken into consideration since these foods are high in total kcals.

Key Points

Athletes who choose to lose weight should do so in the off-season and at a rate of about 1–2 pounds per week. These individuals can achieve an energy deficit via a reduced caloric intake, increased energy expenditure, or both. A key strategy to creating an energy deficit is to consume foods with a low energy density and a high nutrient density while eliminating foods that are energy-dense and nutrient-poor.

Weight Gain in Athletes

There are also athletes seeking to gain weight in an attempt to be more competitive within his or her given sport. Weight gain in the form of increased lean body mass is typically desired. Many athletes believe that if they just eat more (of anything) they can gain weight. While this is true, the additional weight may not be in the form of lean muscle mass.

If an athlete wants to gain muscle mass, strategic nutrition practices can help in the presence of adequate resistance training. In order to minimize gains in fat mass, an athlete needs to be intentional in the practices used to gain muscle mass. Simply drinking "weight gainer" supplements throughout the day may result in excessive calories that will be stored as fat. Ideally, a sports dietitian should be included in the process to provide specific nutrition and training guidelines, but the following information can be helpful for coaches and trainers who may be advising athletes on healthy weight gain strategies.

Athletes should be realistic about weight gain expectations. Important considerations for successful gains in fat-free mass include genetic potential, body frame, and inherent muscle fiber type (individuals who have primarily type II fibers are more likely to experience significant muscle hypertrophy), gender, stage of pubertal growth, rate of weight gain, and training stimulus. Genetics cannot be controlled and some athletes will gain muscle mass much more quickly and to a greater extent than others. Those with a slender frame size (ectomorph) will have less potential to increase muscle mass than will athletes with a larger frame size (meso-morph), and athletes who are "heavy-set" (endomorphs) are also more likely to gain weight but in the form of fat-mass rather than fat-free mass. Mesomorphs are also more likely to have a greater ratio of type II: type I muscle fibers compared to ectomorphs or endomorphs, this further increases the mesomorph's potential for skeletal muscle hypertrophy. In general, males have a greater capacity to increase fat-free mass compared to females; this is due to males' greater release of the anabolic hormone testosterone. Stage of pubertal growth will also be a factor, especially for males. Athletes who have gone through puberty will be more likely to gain muscle mass than will athletes who have not because of increased testosterone production. As with weight loss, rate of weight gain should be gradual and should not exceed 1 pound a week; weight gain at a more rapid rate will likely result in greater fat mass gains. Finally to reiter-ate, training stimulus must be adequate in terms of frequency, duration, and intensity in order to provide the needed overload to induce increases in skeletal muscle protein synthesis. A resistance training program that focuses on a greater number of sets and higher repetitions with lower weights (three to five sets, 8 to 12 reps, ~70 percent of the one repetition maximum) can be useful for muscle hypertrophy and is best facilitated by a coach or athletic trainer.

General nutrition practices for appropriate weight gain include an ex-cess calorie intake of 300 to 500 calories a day and a protein intake of ap-proximately 2.5 g/kg/bw. Increases in caloric intake beyond 500 additional kcals above total daily energy expenditure will likely lead to increases in fat mass because muscle protein synthesis occurs at a relatively slow rate and only so many kcals are needed to optimize muscle building capacity; therefore, kcals above and beyond this amount will be stored as adipose. Additionally, excess kcal consumption in the absence of resistance training will result in increased fat mass because skeletal muscle protein synthesis requires an overload stimulus. Caloric and protein intake should be spread out evenly throughout the day (i.e., five to nine meals and snacks each day and a protein source at each meal and snack). Energy *and* nutrient dense foods should be consumed; see Table 3.3 for examples of appropriate foods. Ergogenic aids and other dietary supplements should be avoided as these products have not been studied in developing athletes and generally do not provide any additional benefit over food-based sources of kcals and protein.

Table 3.3 Energy- and nutrient-dense choices for weight gain

Nuts and seeds (all types)
Avocado
Dried fruits
Whole milk and full fat dairy products
Fatty fish such as salmon
Olive, nut, and avocado oils
Eggs
Whole grain bread and cereal products

Key Points

As with weight loss, many athletes feel pressure to increase body weight and particularly muscle mass to improve their strength and ultimately their performance. Athletes should be aware of limitations to what is attainable including genetic predispositions and body frame size. Athletes seeking increased body mass and specifically muscle mass should consume energy-dense foods, include foods high in protein and healthy sources of fat, and overall should increase their caloric intake by approximately 300 to 500 calories a day.

References and Additional Readings

American Academy of Pediatrics Committee on Sports Medicine and Fitness. 2005. Promotion of healthy weight-control practices in young athletes. *Pediatrics*. 116, no. 6, pp. 1557–1564.

Turocy PS, et al. 2011. National Athletic Trainers' Association position statement: safe weight loss and maintenance practices in sport and exercise. *J Athl Train*. 46, no. 3, pp. 322–336.

CHAPTER 4

Eating Disorders and Disordered Eating

Introduction

Eating disorders are mental health disorders that can be extremely detrimental to physical and psychological well-being. If left untreated, the consequences of these disorders can last a lifetime. Exercise professionals should be able to identify signs and symptoms of disordered eating and eating disorders because early identification leads to earlier treatment, and improves long-term prognosis. The following information is not intended for diagnostic purposes, rather it is intended to help coaches, trainers, and other exercise professionals recognize the unique signs, symptoms, and consequences of various eating disorders as well as how to reduce risk of eating disorders among athletes through fostering healthy eating and training practices.

Classifications of Clinical Eating Disorders

Clinical eating disorders include anorexia nervosa, hallmarked by severe food restriction and excessive weight loss; bulimia nervosa, characterized by a cycle of bingeing and compensatory behaviors such as self-induced vomiting, laxative abuse, and/or excessive exercise; binge eating disorder, defined as recurrent episodes of consuming large quantities of food without compensatory behaviors seen in those with bulimia nervosa; and Other Specified Feeding or Eating Disorder (OSFED), which includes eating and feeding disorders of clinical severity but do not meet the diagnostic criteria of the other three categories. While most exercise professionals do not need to know specific diagnostic criteria, it is important to

be familiar with risks of developing an eating disorder, and able to identify signs and symptoms associated with these life-threatening diseases.

Eating Disorder Risk Factors

Eating disorders and disordered eating are more common among athletes
compared to nonathletic peer groups. Unfortunately, there are many athletes who intentionally engage in unhealthy eating behaviors to achieve a
perceived ideal body weight, or a weight he or she associates with optimal
performance. Any athlete can develop an eating disorder, male or female,
underweight, normal weight, or overweight; coaches and athletic trainers
who only look for potential eating disorder behaviors in low body weight
athletes can potentially misidentify someone who is just naturally thin as
well as miss helping other at-risk athletes.

In general, athletes in weight-sensitive sports are at greatest risk for
developing disordered eating and/or exercise behaviors. Weight-sensitive
sports include those that emphasize a low body weight for a maximum
power-to-weight ratio (distance running, cycling, rock climbing, cross-
country skiing, and ski jumping), those that emphasize aesthetics and
a small physique (gymnastics, figure skating, diving, and various danc-
ing events), and weight-class sports (rowing, weight lifting, wrestling,
and boxing). Athletes in these sports may feel pressure to achieve or
maintain a low body weight because he or she believes it will improve
performance. These pressures may be perceived to come from coaches,
teammates, and/or parents, or may be entirely self-imposed. Other characteristics such as perfectionism, high-achievement orientation, and
early start of sport-specific training are other specific traits, often seen
as positive attributes of an athlete, known to increase risk of disordered
eating behaviors (Sundgot-Borgen et al. 2013). Whatever the source(s),
the pressure to lose excess body fat and/or to maintain a low body weight
can cause occasional dieting efforts to progress into chronic behaviors
that can last a lifetime.

In some weight-class sports there is also a *culture* of accepted extreme *making-weight* practices such as using saunas and excessive exercise to lose water weight or to consume very few calories for several
days prior to a competition. While these behaviors may be temporary,

they increase the risk of an athlete progressing to more chronic dieting behaviors that can promote the development of disordered eating/eating disorders. Exercise professionals and parents can help prevent the adoption of unhealthy eating practices by focusing on athletes' physical performance and health and not excessively focusing on body weight and/or composition. A coach or parent should never encourage an athlete to lose weight, but if an athlete chooses to do so, he or she should be referred to a sports dietitian for an appropriate strategy.

Key Points

Eating disorders are serious and potentially life-threatening conditions that include anorexia nervosa, bulimia nervosa, binge eating disorder, and other specified feeding or eating disorders. Athletes are at greater risk than their nonathletic peers, and weight-dependent sport athletes are particularly at risk. Parents and coaches should not base risk off of weight alone as athletes of all body shapes can struggle with an eating disorder.

Eating Disorder Signs and Symptoms

Disordered eating behaviors can be viewed on a spectrum of dietary and exercise behaviors. On one end of the spectrum are behaviors that allow for healthy and balanced eating and training habits as well as an overall sense of comfort with food, exercise, and one's body. Individuals whose behaviors fall on this end of the spectrum consume adequate calories to meet their energy needs for training and overall health and have a healthy relationship with food. The opposite end of this spectrum includes behaviors such as severe restriction of caloric intake, fasting, eliminating certain food groups from the diet, self-induced vomiting, and excessive exercise intended to compensate for real or perceived overconsumption of calories. Alone or in combination, these practices can progress into the development of a clinically diagnosed eating disorder. Somewhere within the mid-section of the eating disorder spectrum are behaviors that are not necessarily indicative of an eating disorder but, taken too far, can become problematic; such behaviors include engaging in fad diets, repeated weight cycling, compromised body image, and having an excessive preoccupation with food, body weight, and exercise.

Specific eating disorders have unique and identifiable characteristics. In the case of anorexia nervosa, individuals have an intense fear of gaining weight and become obsessed with maintaining a low body weight. Other characteristics of this disorder include dramatic weight loss (or failure to gain weight during a period of growth), preoccupation with food and its contents (i.e., calories, fat grams, carbohydrates, and added sugars), preoccupation with one's weight, and an unrealistic perception of actual body size (i.e., *feeling* fat). Eating-related anxieties and desire to hide atypical eating behaviors may also lead to social isolation, thereby intensifying associated behaviors. Bulimia nervosa includes warning signs such as frequent fluctuations in body weight, avoidance of food-related social events, making highly critical comments regarding body shape and size, and evidence of vomiting behaviors including frequent trips to the restroom after eating, and swollen parotid glands around the cheeks. Individuals who suffer from bulimia report a sense of lack of control over eating and may consume extremely large amounts of food in a short period of time which is followed by self-induced vomiting, excessive laxative use, and/or excessive exercise. Individuals with bulimia nervosa can remain undiagnosed for long periods of time because they do not look emaciated and related behaviors are hidden because of intense shame regarding binging and purging habits. Physical symptoms to look for include swelling of the cheeks or jaw area, calluses on the back of the hands and knuckles, and tooth erosion. Signs and symptoms of binge eating disorder include those associated with bulimia nervosa (i.e., eating large amounts of food in a short period of time, feeling a loss of sense of control over one's eating, and secretive eating behaviors), but there is no evidence of compensatory behaviors and binging behaviors are accompanied by excessive weight gain. If any of these warning signs are identified, an individual should be referred to an expert for further assessment and treatment options.

Consequences of Eating Disorders

Behaviors associated with eating disorders can have dangerous health-related complications. A common complication of self-induced dehydration, purging, excessive laxative use, and/or severe caloric restriction includes clinical electrolyte imbalances which result in irregular heartbeats and possibly heart failure and death. Dehydration can also result in heat exhaustion or even heat stroke which ultimately can be life-threatening, and even moderate dehydration can reduce cardiovascular capacity and ability to thermoregulate. Self-induced vomiting can result in inflammation and potential rupture of the esophagus; and laxative abuse can result in chronic constipation. Individuals with anorexia nervosa often experience slowed heart rate (<55 beats per minute) and very low blood pressure (<100/60 mm Hg) due to hypothalamic-induced reductions in sympathetic nervous system output. Extreme self-starvation can eventually result in heart failure. Even moderate caloric restriction among teenage girls can cause decreased hormonal output which causes a reduction in peak bone mineral density and increases risk of bone injury and ultimately osteoporosis.

Proper nutrition and hydration practices are essential for growing athletes in particular because unhealthy eating habits can delay pubertal development and ultimately may stunt growth, physical maturation, and peak bone density. In a chronically undernourished athlete, maximal force production, power production, speed, mental acuity, and agility are impaired. Not only does performance suffer but the overall health of the athlete is compromised. Chronically undernourished athletes are at risk for nutrient deficiencies, chronic fatigue, increased incidence of illness and infection, anemia, muscle atrophy, general weakness, fainting, and intolerance to cold. Many athletes with prolonged patterns of disordered eating may fail to achieve peak height and bone mass and could face other risks including chronic injuries and stress fractures. These disorders should not be taken lightly and need to be addressed immediately once identified.

Prevention and Treatment of Eating Disorders

Early identification and early treatment of eating disorders and/or eating disorder behaviors is essential for successful long-term recovery. Ideally all eating disorder behaviors could be prevented through fostering a healthy environment and good self-esteem, but in susceptible individuals, prevention tactics may not prove effective. If and when issues do arise, early intervention is of the utmost importance for the individual as well as for the team as there is evidence to suggest that disordered eating behaviors can be socially *contagious*.

Athletes identified as having an eating disorder should be considered an *injured athlete* and should not participate in sport while engaging in unhealthy eating behaviors. In order to return to training and competition, the athlete should be medically cleared by a doctor as well as commit to an eating disorder treatment plan. Such a plan includes working with a sports physician to address any medical concerns, a registered dietitian (ideally a sports dietitian) to ensure adequate energy intake, a licensed psychologist or psychiatrist (preferably one who specializes in eating disorders) to work through psychological causes of the eating disorder, and possibly an exercise specialist or physical therapist if existing injuries are present.

Even when an individual reaches an acceptable body weight or ceases to engage in eating disorder-related behaviors, underlying feelings of inadequacies and anxiety are likely to linger. Relapse is common among those who suffer from eating disorders and is most likely to occur in the midst of dramatic life-changing events. To prevent relapse, underlying mental health conditions must also be treated in order to ensure long-term recovery as evidence suggests that the vast majority of those who are diagnosed also suffer from other mental disorders such as depression, obsessive compulsive disorder, attention-deficit/hyperactivity disorder (ADHD), and bipolar disorder. Often treatment of an eating disorder is a long journey with bumps and setbacks along the road to recovery.

Key Points

Coaches, parents, and staff who work with athletes should be familiar with the signs and symptoms of disordered eating and eating disorders, as well as the health consequences related to eating disorders. Athletes who have been identified with disordered eating or an eating disorder should be referred to a treatment team that at minimum consists of a sports physician, sports dietitian, and therapist.

The Female Athlete Triad

The *female athlete triad* is an increasingly common condition in female athletes. The Triad is a cluster of symptoms that include inadequate energy intake (also known as inadequate energy availability) with or without an eating disorder, missed menstrual cycles (also called amenorrhea), and decreased bone density. It is important to understand that low energy availability, that is, inadequate energy intake, is the cornerstone of the Triad and is what causes the other two components. Adequate energy availability means that an athlete is consuming enough calories to meet her energy demands for sport, activities of daily living, and basic metabolic functions such as respiration, circulation, digestion, and reproduction. If a female athlete has low energy availability because of restricted energy intake or very high levels of physical activity, the body will respond by decreasing estrogen production, thereby decreasing likelihood of a pregnancy for which there is no energy to support. Low estrogen production is evidenced by missed menstrual cycles, delayed menarche, and/or amenorrhea. Decreases in estrogen have also been associated with decreases in bone mass and/or lower peak bone density. This is especially troubling because low energy intake is often found in conjunction with low nutrient intake which further decreases osteoblast (bone-building) activity and causes an even lower peak bone mineral density. While not all female athletes have all three components of the Triad, even having one component indicates a strong likelihood of risk for or presence of the other two Triad members, even if not yet apparent. Thus, identifying an athlete that has one component and providing treatment can prevent the progression of the other two components. See Figure 4.1 for a schematic of the female athlete triad.

It is important to note that in some female athletes, low energy availability results from intentional restrictive intake intended to facilitate achieving or maintaining a low body weight for performance reasons. However, there are also athletes who are simply unaware of their energy needs (how many calories their bodies actually require to support health and exercise) and underconsume calories without intentionally restricting intake. Thus, the female athlete Triad may or *may not* include disordered eating or an eating disorder. Regardless, in either scenario, the cornerstone of treatment for the Triad will include increasing caloric

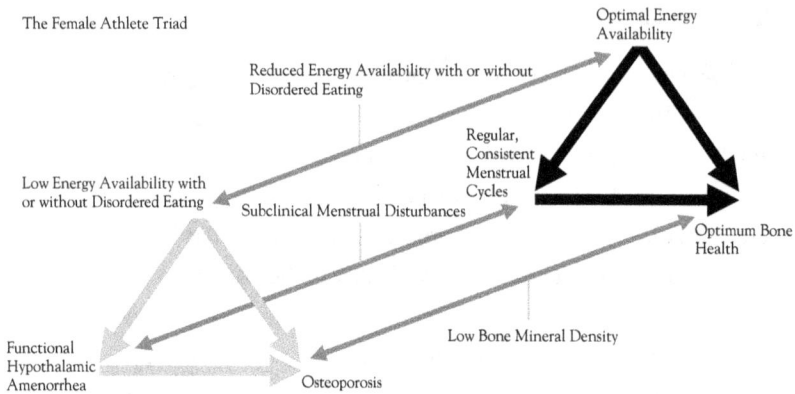

The Female Athlete Triad

Optimal Energy Availability

Reduced Energy Availability with or without Disordered Eating

Regular, Consistent Menstrual Cycles

Low Energy Availability with or without Disordered Eating

Subclinical Menstrual Disturbances

Optimum Bone Health

Functional Hypothalamic Amenorrhea

Osteoporosis

Low Bone Mineral Density

Figure 4.1 Female Athlete Triad Spectrum Schemata.

intake, reducing energy expenditure, or a combination of both. Increased energy intake and/or reduced energy expenditure allows for positive energy availability, which will help stimulate estrogen production, and thus improve menstrual dysfunction and possibly bone mineral density.

Bottom line: When a young woman is not consuming enough energy (kcals) and micronutrients (vitamins and minerals) to meet the energy demand of physical activity and normal biological functioning, she will experience a decrease in estrogen production *which sets the stage for stress fractures now and osteoporosis later*. Female athletes with the Triad also experience more overuse injuries and have lower immune function compared to their healthy peers. If an athlete is experiencing symptoms associated with the female athlete triad it is important to speak to a physician and a sports dietitian as soon as possible, as it may be a sign of a serious eating disorder and girls with eating disorders are at risk for serious and possibly irreversible bone loss.

It is important to note that while females are at greater risk for eating disorders and disordered eating, these eating patterns can also be seen among male athletes. For obvious reasons, the female athlete triad does not apply to males; however, low energy available *is* seen among some male athletes, particularly endurance athletes (cyclists), gravitational athletes (such as ski jumpers), and athletes in sports with weight classes. Although research in this area is sparse and further study is needed to fully understand the repercussions of low energy available among male athletes, we can assume that it increases risk for poor bone mineralization and possibly alters endocrine function. Importantly this includes reduced testosterone output which adversely affects the ability to gain muscle mass and recover from intense exercise. Treatment for male athletes with low energy availability include similar treatment approaches for women; increasing energy intake along with psychological counseling and medical management.

Key Points

As a health and fitness professional, it is important to help young athletes understand that not consuming enough energy (calories) or fluids can be very detrimental to performance. Eating disorders and disordered eating can have severe effects on performance and overall health. Exercise professionals can help prevent eating disorder behaviors by focusing on overall health, not an athlete's weight, and should refrain from commenting on an athlete's body weight. Athletes who are identified as having an eating disorder should be considered *injured* and only allowed to return to sport upon medical clearance and commitment to treatment of their eating disorder. Females are at a greater risk of developing eating disorders which are often associated with the female athlete triad. This is a serious condition that increases risk of stress fractures and poor bone development which leads to osteoporosis later in life.

References and Additional Readings

Beals KA. 2004. *Disordered Eating Among Athletes: A Comprehensive Guide for Health Professionals, 1ˢᵗ edition.* Champaign, IL. Human Kinetics.

Female Athlete Triad Coalition. http://www.femaleathletetriad.org/

National Eating Disorders Association. http://www.nationaleatingdisorders.org/

Sundgot-Borgen J, et al. 2013. How to minimise the health risks to athletes who compete in weight-sensitive sports review and position statement on behalf of the Ad Hoc Research working group on body composition, health and performance, under the auspices of the IOC Medical Commission. *Br J Sports Med.* 47, no. 16, pp. 1012–1022.

CHAPTER 5

Supplements and Ergogenic Aids

Introduction

All competitive athletes are in search of methods to improve performance. Training, nutrition, and rest play key roles, but many athletes choose supplements in an attempt to increase power, speed, strength, size, endurance, or fat loss. However, athletes should be aware that no supplement can replace a nutritious, balanced diet. In general, a foods first, supplements second approach should be taken, and athletes are encouraged to consume a balanced, varied diet that will provide them with needed key nutrients.

All too often athletes rely upon dietary supplements to meet their nutrient needs and pay little attention to the inclusion of important nutrient-rich foods. A nutrient-rich diet that contains foods with a variety of vitamins, minerals, fiber, and the appropriate amount of macronutrients has many beneficial health effects in addition to performance benefits. However, there are certain circumstances when dietary supplements can be appropriate, and these products may complement a whole foods-based diet. As an example, there are situations when a multivitamin may be warranted and there are times when sports nutrition products may support performance.

Ergogenic Aids Defined

The term *ergogenic aid* refers to anything that supposedly improves sport performance above levels anticipated under normal conditions. This includes mechanical ergogenics, such as cleats or clap skates; psychological ergogenics, such as mental imagery; and pharmacological and nutritional ergogenics. In this chapter we use the term in reference to substances consumed with the intent of improving sport performance. The world of nutritional ergogenic aids is vast and diverse and includes everything from sports drinks and energy bars to banned herbal products such as ephedra and even anabolic steroids.

Many supposed ergogenic supplements, despite claims and anecdotal evidence, or "in-house research," do not improve performance and may actually be harmful. Specific to the developing athlete, there are no rigorous scientific studies that examine the long-term consequences of dietary supplement consumption on health, growth and development, or performance; nor is there research to support the effectiveness of nutritional ergogenics among this population. Adolescent athletes may be particularly susceptible to buying into the claims of nutritional ergogenics and should be educated about the inherent risks of supplement consumption.

Regulation of Nutritional Supplements and Ergogenics

Nonfood, nutritional supplements are regulated very differently than prescription drugs. They are not standardized and *do not* have to be proven to be safe or effective before they are put on the market. If a product or substance is proven to be *unsafe* by the Food and Drug Administration, it is taken off the market but this typically requires several incidences of adverse reactions to a given supplement. This is one reason why new, fad supplements can be especially dangerous and possibly detrimental to performance. Caveat emptor!

Manufacturers of supplements are required to have a supplement facts label on the retail packaging, but testing for verification of product contents is voluntary. The actual product may have different ingredients from what is actually claimed. Active ingredients found within the product may not be present in the amounts claimed, and/or contaminated with glass, toxins, lead or other heavy metals, feces, or even unlisted banned substances. If a substance is banned it means that a sporting body has prohibited its use and if found in the blood or urine of an athlete, he or she can be permanently suspended from all forms of professional, collegiate, and Olympic competition. Even supplements and ergogenics bought at the local grocery or drug store may be banned; just because a supplement can legally be purchased does not ensure that it is not banned by a given sporting authority. "Buyer beware" or "caveat emptor" applies directly to the poorly regulated supplement arena. In fact, anabolic steroids, along with ephedrine and caffeine, are one of the most commonly found contaminants in dietary supplements (Petroczi et al., 2011). Although caffeine is legal, ephedra and anabolic steroids certainly are not! For a more inclusive list of banned substances, visit the websites of United States Anti-Doping Agency (USADA) and World Anti-Doping Agency (WADA).

Given these concerns, many governing bodies including the American Academy of Pediatrics Committee on Sports Medicine and Fitness and the International Olympic Committee caution against encouraging young athletes to consume dietary supplements for performance enhancement. In general, dietary supplements should be considered with caution. Education is key, and while many athletes may feel pressure from their peers, coaches, family members, and the media, it is best to consult a sports dietitian or a physician before taking any supplement other than a standard multivitamin. The associated costs and benefits need to be considered before taking a dietary supplement. For example, if an athlete with optimal iron stores chooses to take an iron supplement, he or she will not experience any performance or health benefit but may suffer from stomach upset, constipation, decreased calcium absorption, and a thinner wallet.

Key Points

Before taking any supplement, ask your sport dietitian or physician the following:

- Are they safe?
- Do they work?
- Are they banned?

Categorizing Supplements and Ergogenics

Because dietary supplements include such a wide variety of products, it is helpful to divide them into different categories to examine risk and efficacy. A basic supplement categorization outline as well as examples from each category can be found in Table 5.1.

Category 1 Supplements

Many of the Category 1 supplements can help athletes achieve nutritional goals during intense training, extended workouts, or competition and have minimal risk for adverse health effects. Supplements from this category provide an alternative to whole foods, which might be impractical to eat immediately before or during intense exercise. The following information provides basic recommendations for use of these products, though always refer to a sports dietitian for further questions regarding individual use. See Table 5.1 for an outline of Category 1 supplements.

Vitamin and Mineral Supplements

Multivitamins/minerals. Multivitamins/minerals represent the most commonly consumed dietary supplements among adolescents and adults. Some of these supplements include an array of both vitamins and minerals while others only contain vitamins. Multivitamin/mineral supplementation may be recommended for athletes who consume low-calorie diets, are extremely fussy and only eat limited types of foods, have allergies to many different kinds of foods, or have a medical condition that increases the need for specific nutrients. There are also athletes who, for a variety of reasons, restrict intake of specific food groups (i.e., vegan athletes who do not consume any animal products) and can also benefit from multivitamin/mineral supplementation.

Multivitamin/mineral supplements cannot replace a balanced, nutrient-rich diet, nor will a multivitamin/mineral improve athletic performance unless there is a preexisting nutrient deficiency. Some athletes may receive a false sense of security by taking a multivitamin/mineral and believe it can take the place of consuming fresh fruits and vegetables and other nutrient-rich foods; however, there are many other components in fruits, vegetables, and seeds that offer important physiological benefits and should be consumed regularly regardless of supplement use.

When a multivitamin/mineral supplement is warranted, the current recommendation is to choose a general over-the-counter supplement with a broad array of essential nutrients and no more than 100 percent of the daily Dietary Reference Intake (DRI). Athletes should avoid multivitamin and mineral supplements that contain excessive amounts of any given nutrient; for example, some supplements with the marketing claim of improving energy metabolism contain upward of 1,000 percent of the DRI for B_{12} and other B vitamins; this is unnecessary and the long-term effects of such high doses are not well known.

Calcium.   *Calcium* is essential for proper bone mineralization (i.e., hardening). The importance of calcium intake during adolescence and young adulthood is underscored by the fact that calcium deposition in the bone is about four times greater than in adulthood. However, many athletes do not consume adequate calcium. Athletes of particular risk include those with low caloric intake or who are on restrictive diets, those who avoid dairy-containing foods (a major source of calcium in the diet), or those with malabsorption issues such as celiac disease.

Daily calcium requirement for children and adolescents aged 9 to 18 years is approximately 1,300 mg. Children and adolescents who chronically consume inadequate amounts of calcium risk failing to reach optimal peak bone mass by their late 20s and increased risk for osteoporosis later in life. Because of these long-term consequences, it is particularly important to educate athletes on the importance of adequate calcium consumption, and athletes should be provided guidance on how to increase their consumption of calcium-rich foods on a daily basis. Excellent sources of calcium include dairy foods (milk, yogurt, and cheese), dairy alternatives (calcium-fortified soy and almond milk), leafy green vegetables, and tofu.

If an athlete is unable to consume adequate amounts of calcium from food sources, calcium supplements can be used to meet the recommended 1,300 mg/day intake. Calcium carbonate and calcium citrate are most common (calcium citrate being preferable for someone with acid reflux disease) and are generally well-tolerated. Calcium supplements are best absorbed in 500 mg doses, so if greater amounts are needed (such as

1,000 mg/day) then 500 mg doses should be taken at two different times during the day. Avoid taking calcium with iron or foods high in iron, as one impairs the absorption of the other.

Vitamin D.   Vitamin D, also known as the sun vitamin because it can be produced via cutaneous synthesis with adequate duration and intensity of sun exposure, is essential for calcium absorption in the body. Therefore, inadequate consumption results in poor bone mineralization. Vitamin D also likely plays a role in skeletal muscle and immune function. Current daily recommended intake for adolescent athletes is 600 IU. Vitamin D is found in few food sources, though moderate amounts can be consumed from fish (especially salmon and tuna), and vitamin D-fortified dairy and soy products such as milk and soy milk. Unfortunately, vitamin D deficiency is quite common among young athletes, especially those who train inside and have minimal sun exposure. Also at greater risk of vitamin D deficiency are athletes with darker skin tone, those living at higher latitudes, and those with malabsorption issues. If there is any question regarding deficiency, an athlete can easily have vitamin D status assessed by his or her doctor via blood testing. Based on results, supplementation may be recommended; specific dosing should be provided by a physician or sports dietitian.

Iron.   *Iron* is an important mineral because it is a component of hemoglobin which helps transport oxygen throughout the body. Oxygen is required by almost every cell in the body and allows for the continued resynthesis of the ATP required to sustain cellular and organism life. Low iron intake can impair synthesis of hemoglobin and reduces oxygen transport. Poor oxygen transport causes feelings of extreme fatigue, weakness, and shortness of breath, all of which can potentially result in a deterioration in performance. Daily recommended iron intake is 10 mg for children 4 to 8 years; 8 mg for ages 9 to 13 years, and 11 mg and 15 mg for males and females, respectively, ages 14 to 18 years. Men and women over the age of 18 require approximately 8 and 18 mg/day, women have higher iron needs due to losses associated with monthly menstrual cycles. Dietary sources of iron include meat (particularly red meat), legumes, leafy green vegetables, tofu, and fortified cereals and grains.

While many athletes consume adequate sources of dietary iron, certain athletes risk inadequate intake and may benefit from iron supplementation. Vegetarian athletes, endurance athletes, female athletes, and athletes on restrictive/low-calorie diets have an increased risk of iron deficiency anemia. If anemia is suspected, iron status should be assessed before initiating supplementation. In addition to traditional iron status tests, serum ferritin should be checked as this is a more sensitive measure of iron status. If supplementation is warranted, it is best to consult a physician or sports dietitian for appropriate dosage since the degree of deficiency determines the recommended amount of supplementation. Consuming foods with vitamin C enhances iron absorption and co-consumption of foods high in vitamin C, such as orange juice, is recommended. If larger doses of iron are warranted (60 mg/day or more), twice-daily supplementation may help minimize gastrointestinal side effects.

Sports Nutrition Products

Sports nutrition products most commonly include sports drinks, sports bars, and sports gels. In general these supplements carry a very low risk for banned substance contamination and negligible side effects. These products may be appropriate in specific athletic contexts depending upon the sport type and duration of activity and can be consumed immediately prior to, during, and/or immediately following long-duration (>60 to 90 minutes) physical activity. Most sports nutrition products are specifically formulated to contain the appropriate amount and types of carbohydrate for optimal absorption and typically provide electrolytes (namely sodium) to help replace any sweat-related losses. Given the importance of carbohydrate consumption during longer and higher-intensity activities, bars, gels, drinks and other products have a useful application and their portability makes them especially convenient. Furthermore, there is evidence to support the use of sport drinks as a means to improve performance during extended exercise as well as to rehydrate and replenish muscle glycogen stores postexercise.

While sports nutrition products such as bars, gels, and sports drinks should not make up the foundation of an athlete's diet, the portability and convenience of these products make them a practical option for meeting nutrient needs before, during, and after training. Athletes who may benefit from consumption of these products include those with heavy training volumes, those trying to increase muscle mass, athletes experiencing rapid growth, and athletes who need portable food options due to training and traveling schedules. However, drinking sports drink while watching television is not the appropriate application of this product.

Protein powders

Protein powders, as with all dietary supplements, are poorly regulated and have a higher risk for contamination than do sports drinks, bars, and gels. Heavy metals such as lead, arsenic, and cadmium, and other ingredients including anabolic steroids have been found as contaminants. Furthermore, through third party analysis, some protein powders have been found to contain far less protein and much more carbohydrate filler than what is stated on the packaging label. Unfortunately, as evidenced by the high use of these products among 12- to 18-year-olds, adolescent athletes are especially susceptible to marketing claims advertised on protein powders. Developing athletes can easily meet protein needs through inclusion of protein-rich food sources including Greek yogurt, cottage cheese and other dairy foods; lean meats and fish; eggs; nuts and seeds; beans; and soy-containing foods such as tofu and edamame. A smoothie made with Greek yogurt and milk can have just as much protein as a shake made with protein powder!

There are circumstances when it may be acceptable for certain athletes to consume protein powders. Examples include athletes who are restricting caloric intake and thus have higher protein needs, athletes with very high calorie needs (such as 4,000 to 6,000 calories a day), and athletes aiming to increase lean body mass. While these athletes can meet their calorie and protein needs with food, protein supplements represent a convenient adjunct to a nutrient-rich diet. In these cases, consumption of whey protein (hydrolyzed whey or whey isolate) powders have been shown to be effective in maintaining and increasing lean body mass. Athletes should look for products that have a third-party quality control assurance to verify the product contains what is stated on the label.

Judicious intake is important as adolescent athletes may be prone to the "more is better" mentality and if one scoop is good, four is better. This is not the case, and athletes should be cautioned against excessive consumption of anything, particularly dietary supplements.

Key Points

Category 1 supplements overall are relatively safe for consumption, though supplements such as protein powders have a higher rate of contamination and should be consumed with caution. Multivitamins and individual vitamin and mineral supplements cannot replace a balanced, whole foods-based diet, though there are circumstances when their usage may be warranted to prevent deficiency. Sports nutrition products including sports bars, gels, and drinks, when used appropriately, may assist an athlete in meeting their nutrient needs before, during, and after exercise and thus may support optimal performance.

Category 2 Supplements

Category 2 supplements have some evidence to support physiological benefits; however, these supplements have an increased risk of negative side effects, such as upset stomach, diarrhea, and/or potential malabsorption of other nutrients, all of which can interfere with training and performance. Category 2 supplements also carry a higher risk of containing illegal/banned substances. There is little to no research to support the use of these products among developing athletes since research studies on individuals under 18 years of age is typically considered unethical. Thus, what may be safe for an adult athlete may not be safe for the growth and development of a younger athlete.

Prior to use of Category 2 products, it is prudent to seek the advice of a sports dietitian to ensure the product is safe, effective, and of the highest quality. Furthermore, these products work only when used appropriately (i.e., in the correct dosage and for the intended purpose). For example, most young athletes would never have the need to take glucosamine because it is intended to reduce the pain associated with arthritis and, in the case of creatine supplementation, cross-country runners would benefit little because of the associated increases in water weight. Just because a product has the potential to improve an aspect of sport performance does not justify its use among all athletes.

Among Category 2 supplements, caffeine is likely the most widely used and accepted. Caffeine can be found in coffee, teas, soda, as well as the increasingly popular varieties of *energy drinks*. Products such as Red Bull, Monster, and Full Throttle are especially popular among high-school and collegiate athletes. Younger athletes can be especially susceptible to the marketing ploys of these products and most are endorsed by famous athletes and celebrities. These drinks bring promises of endless energy and improved performance but all individuals and especially developing athletes should be cautioned against the use of these products. These products contain substances in addition to caffeine, such as gaurana and taurine, which are understudied and unregulated. Additionally third-party product analysis has found the amount of caffeine in these products is often higher than what is listed on the label (*if* the caffeine content is noted at all). Because adolescents are more likely to overconsume these drinks (i.e., drink several at one time), this population is also at an increased risk for experiencing adverse effects, such as liver and kidney damage, agitation, seizures, elevated heart rate, cardiac dysrhythmias, and possibly cardiac arrest and death. There is even evidence to suggest an increased incidence of risky behaviors and increase risk of injury after energy drink consumption.

When discussing energy drinks with adolescent athletes, it is helpful to point out that energy drinks have very little scientific evidence to support any ergogenic effect but have well-documented adverse side effects. Why would an athlete select such a product when there are other beverages available, namely sports drinks, which have been scientifically shown to improve performance? Adolescent athletes may not be as concerned for their health and the long-term consequences associated with energy drink consumption, but quite often they *do* care about their performance. Highlighting the performance benefits associated with sports drink consumption may serve to impact their beverage choices.

Category 3 Supplements

Category 3 substances include most herbal products, ergogenic pharmaceuticals, and supplements not listed in Categories 1 and 2. This category

Table 5.1 *Categorization of nutritional and dietary supplements*

Category 1 Supplements Generally Considered to Be Safe and Effective	Category 2 Supplements with Potential to Enhance Performance	Category 3 Supplements with Unfounded Claims and Banned Substances
1. Contain nutrients in amounts similar to levels specified in DRIs and similar to the amounts found in food 2. Provide a convenient and practical way to increase nutrient intake during training 3. Are generally acknowledged as safe and valuable products by sports medicine and science experts	1. Contain nutrients or other food components in amounts greater than the DRIs or typically provided by foods 2. Claim to enhance sports performance through a pharmacological or physiological effect 3. Some evidence exists for these products but individual results will vary and benefits may be sport-specific 4. Should be used only under the direction of an appropriate sports medicine/science practitioner	1. Despite claims, no scientific proof of beneficial effects or products are illegal/banned. Products are at high risk of contamination or mislabeling. 2. May contain substances that could lead to a positive drug test
Examples: Sport drinks, sport gels, sport bars, liquid meal supplements, whey protein, multivitamin/mineral, iron, and calcium supplements not exceeding DRIs	*Examples:* Creatine, caffeine, beetroot juice, bicarbonate, B-alanine, branch chain amino acids, individual amino acids, glucosamine, fish oils	*Examples:* Herbals and supplements not listed in Category 1 or 2 (such as ephedra and supplements that are not proven to be free of illegal substances), and banned over-the-counter medications and pharmaceuticals

includes all products that are illegal, banned, or are likely to be contaminated with banned substances. Category 3 supplements also include products that have little or no scientific evidence to support safety and efficacy. These products may use testimonials from athletes and celebrities to support performance-enhancing claims. Anecdotal claims should never be used in place of rigorous scientific inquiry as a means to determine safety and efficacy! Because of the high-risk-to-low-benefit ratio, Category 3 substances should not be used under any circumstances.

Key Points

In the end, the athlete is responsible for what he or she puts into his or her body. It is important to research products thoroughly prior to consumption and always be skeptical of lofty claims. Under most circumstances, consuming nutrient-rich foods is a better approach to meet micro- and macronutrient needs. Many claimed ergogenics lack sufficient evidence to be considered true ergogenics.

Additional Resources

Since dietary supplements represent a very complex and ever-evolving topic of great interest to athletes of all ages and abilities, the following reputable references provide in-depth and reliable information on a variety of supplements.

The Australian Institute of Sport provides "Fact Sheets" for different supplements and a useful supplement classification system: http://www .ausport.gov.au/ais/nutrition/supplements/classification

The US Anti-Doping Agency (USADA) website provides the most up-to-date information on illegal and banned substances as well as a "Supplement 411" online tutorial: http://www.usada.org/

The World Anti-Doping Agency (WADA) website provides valuable information as well as the annually updated, Prohibited List, "which identifies the substances and methods prohibited to athletes in- and out-of-competition." https://www.wada-ama.org/

The Gatorade Sports Science Institute's website includes current information and research articles on sports nutrition supplements:

http://www.gssiweb.org/en

The National Institute on Drug Abuse through the National Institutes of Health offers information on drugs of abuse including information on the health risks of anabolic steroid use:

https://www.drugabuse.gov/drugs-abuse/steroids-anabolic

References and Additional Readings

Ferrando AA, et al. 2010. Essential amino acids for muscle protein accretion. *Strength Cond J.* 32, no. 1, pp. 87–92.

Fink HH, et al. 2013. *Practical Applications in Sports Nutrition*. Burlington, MA. Jones & Bartlett Publishers.

Petroczi A, et al. 2011. Mission impossible? Regulatory and enforcement issues to ensure safety of dietary supplements. *Food Chem Toxicol,* 49, pp. 393–402.

Saunders MJ, et al. 2007. Consumption of an oral carbohydrate-protein gel improves cycling endurance and prevents postexercise muscle damage. *J Strength Cond Res.* 21, no. 3, pp. 678–684.

Shimomura Y, et al. 2004. Exercise promotes BCAA catabolism: effects of BCAA supplementation on skeletal muscle during exercise. *J Nutrition.* 134, no. 6, pp. 1583S–1587S.

Ziegenfuss TN, et al. 2010. Protein for sports: new data and new recommendations. *Strength Cond J.* 32, no. 1, pp. 65–70.

CHAPTER 6

Recipes for Athletes and Additional Resources

Introduction

This text has provided education on *what* developing athletes should be eating, *when* they should be eating, and practical tips and suggestions for *how* to make this happen. This chapter takes the *how* one step further by offering easy, convenient, balanced, and delicious recipes. These recipes are simple enough to be prepared by the novice cook, and are nutrient dense, which means they are packed with vitamins, minerals, and good sources of carbohydrates, proteins, and fats. Best of all, these recipes are great tasting. There are breakfast, lunch, and dinner recipes as well as recipes for sauces, sweets, and snacks. Finally, the chapter concludes with a list of reputable websites and resources for additional sports nutrition information.

Breakfast Recipes

Convenience Store Breakfast

- One banana
- 16 ounce low-fat strawberry or chocolate milk
- Clifbar

Crunch-Time Breakfast (also great for post-Workouts)
- 1 cup 1 percent milk, soymilk, or yogurt
- 1 scoop protein powder (such as soy or whey protein)
- One frozen banana and/or ½ cup frozen berries
- 1 to 2 tbsp wheat germ
- Three to four ice cubes

Put all in a blender and pour into a to-go container.

Power Muffins
- 1 cup all-purpose flour
- 1 cup nonfat dry milk
- ½ tsp salt
- 2 tsp baking powder
- 1 tsp nutmeg
- 2 tsp cinnamon
- 2 cups pumpkin (fresh or canned)
- Two eggs or equivalent egg substitute
- 1 cup raisins or craisins
- ½ cup brown sugar
- 1 tbsp vanilla extract
- 2 tbsp butter (melted)

Preheat oven to 375° Fahrenheit. Grease muffin tins. Pour boiling water over raisins and allow them to soak until plump; drain off excess fluid and pat dry. Combine dry ingredients in medium-sized bowl. Combine wet ingredients in large bowl. Add dry mixture and raisins to the wet mixture. Combine with floured hands; mixture will be sticky. Do not overmix. With clean hands, ball up dough and place in muffin tins. Bake for 30 to 35 minutes. Muffins will be quite moist and pudding-like on the inside. Cook longer for less-moist muffins.

Yield: 16 muffins

Power Breakfast Cereal
- ½ cup whole oats
- ½ cup 1 percent milk (or soy milk)
- One egg
- Half banana, ½ cup frozen berries, or ¼ cup dried fruit
- Walnuts or other nuts as topping
- Brown sugar or honey (optional)

Place the oats, milk, egg, and any frozen fruit in a microwave-safe bowl and mix well. Microwave on high for 1 minute, stir, and microwave for an additional minute. Let it sit for 1 minute, top with dried fruit, nuts, and add additional milk or sweetener if desired.

Standard Scrambled Eggs
- Three eggs or one egg and three egg whites
- 1 oz mozzarella cheese
- Green pepper, red pepper, onion, frozen vegetable mix (or fresh!)
- Salsa
- Tabasco sauce

Microwave the frozen veggies on high for 3 to 4 minutes; drain off any excess water. Scramble the eggs and mix in the veggies and cheese. Top with salsa, fresh tomatoes, and/or an additional sprinkling of cheese. If using fresh vegetables, dice and sauté with a little olive oil in a separate pan.

Serve this meal with two pieces of whole-grain bread and a bowl of fresh fruit.

Or put it in a large whole wheat tortilla for a to-go complete breakfast (also excellent for lunch and dinner).

Breakfast Tacos (Recipe Credit: Kristi Spence)
- Three eggs
- ¼ cup skim milk or water
- ¼ tsp salt
- ¼ tsp pepper
- One medium tomato, chopped
- One handful fresh spinach
- ¼ cup sharp cheddar cheese, shredded
- Two corn or small whole wheat tortillas
- Salsa

Heat nonstick skillet over med–high heat.

In a large bowl, whisk the eggs, milk (or water), salt, and pepper until frothy (~1 minute). Add to the skillet. Just before the eggs finish cooking, add the tomato and spinach. Continue cooking until the tomatoes have softened and the spinach is wilted, ~2 minutes.

Scoop the eggs into the tortillas, top with the cheese and a spoonful of salsa.

Lunch and Dinner Recipes

Cha-Cha Chili
- 2 large cans diced tomatoes
- 1 can red kidney beans
- 1 can black beans
- 1 can garbanzo beans
- 1 lb ground sirloin
- 4 to 6 oz salsa
- 4 oz red wine
- 1 tbsp cumin
- 1 tbsp chili powder (or to taste)
- 1 tbsp black pepper
- 2 tbsp fresh minced garlic
- One large sliced carrot
- One large diced green pepper
- One large diced onion

Brown the sirloin and drain off excess fat. Sauté green pepper, carrot, and onion in a little olive oil and red wine until vegetables are barely tender. Put all in a big pot and let it simmer for a couple of hours. This chili improves overnight and freezes great. Try serving it over the green pepper cornbread.

Yield: 10–a 1 cup servings

Green Pepper Cornbread
- ½ cup whole wheat flour
- ½ cup all-purpose flour
- 1 cup cornmeal
- 2 tsp baking powder
- ½ tsp salt
- 2 tsp black pepper
- 2 tsp red pepper flakes
- Two large eggs

- ¼ cup honey
- ¾ cup plain nonfat yogurt
- ½ cup skim milk
- 1 cup reduced-fat cheddar cheese (shredded)
- 1 can corn
- One large diced green pepper

Preheat oven to 400° Fahrenheit. Mix dry ingredients in a large bowl. Mix wet ingredients, corn, green pepper, and ⅔ cup of cheese in a separate large bowl; reserve ⅓ of the cheese. Add dry ingredients to wet and mix until just combined. Pour batter into a greased bread pan or casserole dish; some extra batter may be left over, use any extras for muffins. Put remaining cheese on top of batter and bake for 45 minutes or until toothpick comes out clean and top of bread is golden brown. Muffins should be baked for 25 minutes at 400° Fahrenheit.

Yield: 12 servings

Veggie Pasta Salad
- 4 oz whole wheat penne pasta
- Two large tomatoes (diced)
- ½ cup fresh basil
- One large broccoli head (cut-up)
- 2 tbsp capers
- 2 tsp fresh garlic (minced)
- 3 oz feta cheese
- 1 tbsp lemon juice
- ¼ cup vegetable broth
- 1 tbsp balsamic vinegar

Cook pasta to *el dente*. Drain and rinse pasta in cold water, place in large bowl. Steam broccoli, allow it to cool and add to pasta. Add remaining ingredients and toss. For some extra protein try adding grilled chicken, fish, or even canned tuna or salmon.

Yield: 4 servings

Annie's Power Mac n' Cheese
- One box of Annie's Mac n' Cheese (any variety)
- One bag of spinach (fresh or frozen and thawed)
- 1 can of diced tomatoes
- 1 can of black beans (or other variety)
- 2 tsp garlic
- Fresh or dried basil
- Salt and pepper to taste

Make the Mac n' Cheese according to the directions. Add the remaining ingredients and stir. The raw spinach will cook down nicely as you stir.

Optional:
In addition to or in place of the beans you can add cooked chicken/steak, canned tuna, ground beef/turkey, or even tofu.

Crock-Pot Chicken
- Chicken, any cut is fine but remove skin and excess fat.
- Potatoes, cubed
- One onion cut into large chunks
- One green or red pepper cut into large chunks
- Rosemary
- Garlic
- 1 tbsp olive oil
- 1 tbsp balsamic vinegar
- 1 tbsp lemon juice
- Salt and pepper to taste

Place all ingredients into crock-pot and cook on low for about 8 hours or on high for 4 hours. Serve this meal with steamed broccoli or a side salad.

Pumped Pizza
- Premade pizza crust (choose one without hydrogenated oils)
- Pasta/pizza sauce (choose one without high-fructose corn syrup)

- Mozzarella cheese
- Feta cheese

Toppings (choose as many as you like):
- Artichoke hearts
- Cooked chicken
- Bell peppers
- Onions
- Spinach
- Tomatoes
- Black beans
- Salsa
- Pineapple
- Basil

Assemble pizza, add toppings, and cook at 400° Fahrenheit until crust and cheese are golden brown.

Serve this meal with a bowl of fresh fruit and cottage cheese.

Stir-fry with Brown Rice
- Brown rice (white rice can be substituted but brown rice has more fiber, protein, vitamins, and minerals)
- Steak, chicken, or pork, precut for stir-fry (shrimp can be used too)
- Fresh ginger grated or 1 tbsp of chopped jar variety
- Two cloves fresh garlic or 2 tsp of chopped jar variety
- Soy sauce or tamari sauce
- Peanut oil (about 2 tsp per serving)
- Sesame oil (about 1 tsp per serving)
- ¼ head red cabbage
- Sugar snap peas
- Red pepper
- Green pepper
- Onion

Other vegetables that stir-fry well:
- Water chestnuts
- Bamboo

- Edamame
- Broccoli
- Bok choy

You can also use a frozen vegetable stir-fry mix (choose one without additives/flavorings)

Cook rice in rice cooker or on stove according to instructions. The rice will take anywhere from 20 to 60 minutes to cook so start it first (brown rice takes longer than white rice).

In a very large skillet, or preferably a wok, heat the peanut oil. When hot, add the meat, ginger, garlic, and onion. Continue to cook for a few minutes then add the peppers, peas, cabbage, sesame oil, and soy sauce. Cook until the vegetables are tender but not soft.

Timing is important with stir-fry. Make sure you add slower cooking vegetables (onions, carrots, and broccoli) and meats first. Chicken needs to be cooked more thoroughly than beef or pork and shrimp does not take very much time at all (and is tough when overcooked). Sesame oil should be added at the end because it is more delicate oil and has the tendency to burn. If you want more flavor, try adding the ginger and garlic later in the cooking process because they will retain more flavor.

Grilled Salmon with Spinach Salad
- Salmon, fresh wild caught (if available)
- Extra-virgin olive oil
- Lemon juice
- Salt and pepper to taste
- Fresh dill

Drizzle oil and lemon juice over salmon (both sides) and grill. Do not overcook! Salt and pepper to taste; top with a lemon wedge and fresh dill. If ambitious, try buying a cedar board (can be found at many grocery stores now) and grill the salmon on it. It adds a very pleasant flavor to the fish.

Spinach Salad
- One bag of spinach
- Strawberries, sliced
- Almonds, sliced or slivers
- Orange or yellow bell pepper, sliced
- Mushrooms, sliced
- Extra-virgin olive oil and white balsamic vinegar for dressing

Serve this meal with leftover rice or pasta (from meal made previously), or with a crusty French or ciabatta bread, or tortillas (they can be grilled with the salmon)

Pasta Sauces with Protein

To any high-quality jarred pasta sauce variety (one without high-fructose corn syrup such as Newman's Own or Wild Oats) add any of the following ingredients:

- Tuna
- Cooked ground beef/turkey
- Leftover chicken
- Cooked spinach
- Black beans (or other variety)
- Cottage cheese
- Mozzarella cheese

Vegetables can also be added to the sauce:

- Diced peppers
- Onions
- Cooked eggplant
- Spinach

Serve this sauce over pasta with steamed broccoli or fresh fruit on the side.

Banana Sushi (Recipe Credit: Kristi Spence)

- Two slices whole wheat bread, crusts removed
- One banana, peeled, ends trimmed
- ¼ cup peanut butter or apple butter

Lay two slices of bread on the counter next to each other, slightly overlapping one another to create one big rectangular piece. Push together at the seam and use a rolling pun to gently flatten the slices of bread.

Gently spread the peanut butter/apple butter evenly over both pieces of bread and lay a whole banana in the middle. Carefully roll up the bread around the banana, bringing one long end over the other. Slice the log into six pieces that are ~1- to 1.5-inch thick and serve!

Yield: serves 1 to 2 people

Spinach Pie (Recipe Credit: Kristi Spence)

- 1 pint low-fat cottage cheese or ricotta cheese
- 1 cup part skim mozzarella cheese, shredded
- ⅓ cup Parmesan cheese, shredded
- Four large eggs
- 10 oz package of frozen, chopped spinach, thawed and well-drained
- One red bell pepper, finely chopped
- 3 tbsp sun-dried tomatoes, chopped
- ½ tsp salt
- ½ tsp pepper

Preheat oven to 350° and spray a 9-inch pie dish with nonstick cooking spray.

Lightly beat eggs in a large bowl. Add all other ingredients and mix well.

Pour mixture into prepared pie dish and bake 50 to 60 minutes or until the top is starting to brown and the mixture is set.

Note: This crustless quiche can also be made in muffin tins and can be frozen for future use.

Yield: 4–6 servings

Tofu Tacos (Recipe Credit: Kristi Spence)

- One block extrafirm tofu, drained
- 1 tbsp + 1 tsp ground cumin
- 1 tbsp + 1 tsp chili powder
- 1 tsp coriander
- 2 tbsp dried oregano
- ½ tsp salt
- 1 tsp crushed red pepper (or less if you are sensitive to spicy food)
- 2 tbsp canola oil, divided
- One yellow onion, diced
- Two medium carrots, peeled and finely chopped
- Three to four roasted red peppers (jarred peppers are a great option!)
- Two cloves garlic, minced
- Three to four leaves of kale, stems removed and chopped
- ½ cup chicken or vegetable broth
- Corn or whole wheat tortillas
- Sharp cheddar cheese, shredded (for topping tacos)
- Salsa (optional)

Drain the tofu by placing it between two plates for ~1 hour. Blot any extra water with paper towels.

Preheat oven to 350°. While tofu drains, mix 1 tbsp each cumin and chili powder, coriander, oregano, salt, crushed red pepper, and 1 tbsp canola oil in a bowl to form a paste.

Slice drained tofu into ¼-inch thick pieces and mix with the spice mixture. Place spiced tofu on a baking sheet and bake ~30 minutes or until crispy on both sides. Remove from the oven and slice any large tofu pieces into strips.

While tofu bakes, heat remaining tablespoon canola oil in a large sauté pan. Add the onion, carrot, 1 tsp each cumin and chili powder and cook until the onion is translucent, ~5 to 7 minutes. Add the pepper and cook until the carrot is soft. Stir in the garlic and baked tofu.

Add the kale with the broth and stir until kale has wilted, ~2 to 3 minutes.

Check for seasonings and salt. Wrap tofu mixture in a slightly toasted tortilla, top with a sprinkle of sharp cheddar cheese and a scoop of salsa, if desired.

Yield: 4 servings

Salmon Salad in Pita Pockets (Recipe Credit: Kristi Spence)

- One large can or pouch of wild salmon (tuna works well also)
- One whole wheat pita pocket, cut in half
- ½ tbsp olive oil
- ½ tbsp balsamic vinegar
- Fresh thyme or parsley
- 2 tbsp grated Parmesan cheese
- One large tomato, sliced
- Salt and pepper, to taste

Drain the salmon if canned and combine with all other ingredients through Parmesan cheese.

Stuff salmon salad into the pita pockets and top with tomato slices.

Yield: 2 servings

Pasta, Pesto, Sun-dried Tomatoes (Recipe Credit: Kristi Spence)

- 1 lb small pasta (preferably whole wheat)
- ⅓–½ cup fresh basil pesto
- ¼ cup chopped sun-dried tomatoes

Cook pasta in a large pot of boiling, salted water until cooked al dente—should be a bit firm to the bite. Drain and toss immediately with pesto and sun-dried tomatoes.

Serve warm, at room temperature, or cold.

Greek Burgers (Recipe Credit: Kristi Spence)

- 1 lb extralean beef, buffalo, or elk
- Two cloves garlic, minced
- 1½ tsp tomato paste
- 1½ tsp dried oregano
- Pinch of salt and pepper, to taste

- 1½ roasted red pepper from a jar, chopped
- 1 tbsp crumbled feta cheese

To serve
- Four slices sharp white cheddar cheese
- Four lettuce leaves
- Whole wheat rolls or English muffins

Mix all ingredients together in a large bowl, taking care not to over-work the meat. Divide into four pieces and shape into patties. Can be stored in fridge until ready to grill.

Grill ~6 minutes each side until burgers are cooked through. When they have about 2 minutes left, lightly toast the buns and add a slice of cheese to the burger.

Top the cooked burger with a splash of Balsamic vinegar and lettuce leaf.

Yield: 4 servings

Ginger Lime Chicken Skewers (Recipe Credit: Kristi Spence)
- Two boneless, skinless chicken breasts cut lengthwise into three strips (you can also use tenders)

For the marinade:
- 1 tbsp canola oil
- ½ tsp crushed red pepper flakes
- 2 tbsp soy sauce
- 1 tsp fresh ginger, minced
- One clove garlic, minced
- Lime juice from one lime

Place a wooden or metal skewer through each chicken strip. Place on a platter or in a plastic container.

Whisk all marinade ingredients together and pour over chicken skewers.

Cover and refrigerate chicken for 1 to 2 hours.

Preheat oven to 350. Roast chicken until cooked through, ~15 minutes. Grilling is also a great option.

Sauces and Sweets

Sour Cream Salsa Dip
- Light sour cream
- Favorite salsa (green or red)

Just mix the two together for a creamy veggie dip with a little kick. Try adding some avocado, garlic, fresh tomato, or shallots to the mix.

Yield: 10 servings

Yogurt–Herb Dip
- 1 cup plain low-fat Greek yogurt
- 1 tbsp balsamic vinegar
- 2 tsp garlic (fresh minced)
- 1 tbsp rosemary
- 1 tbsp brown mustard
- ½ tsp salt

Just mix all up and you are ready to go! Try adding some orange marmalade for an interesting citrus twist. Vary the spices to your liking.

Yield: 10 servings

Peanut Butter Tofu Spread
- 1 tbsp natural peanut butter
- 4 oz soft tofu
- 1 tbsp honey
- 2 tsp cinnamon

Place all ingredients in food processor and mix or mix by hand in small bowl. Try adding different spices and omitting the honey for a more savory sandwich spread/vegetable dip. This dip is also great with jam instead of honey.

Yield: 6 servings

Baked Apples
- Six tart apples
- ¼ cup water
- ¼ cup honey
- ¼ cup brown sugar
- 2 cups plain low-fat yogurt
- 2 tbsp cinnamon
- 2 tsp nutmeg
- 2 tsp cardamom

Core apples and cut into bite-sized pieces (leave skins on), place in baking dish, and add water, brown sugar and spices. Bake at 350° Fahrenheit until apples are tender. Serve immediately in custard dishes, top with yogurt, and drizzle with honey and cinnamon.

Yield: 6 servings

Brown Rice Pudding
- 2 cups cooked brown rice
- 2 cup evaporated nonfat milk (unsweetened)
- One egg
- ½ cup brown sugar
- 1 cup raisins
- 1 tbsp cinnamon
- 1 tbsp cardamom
- 2 tsp almond or vanilla extract
- 1 tsp salt
- 2 tbsp butter

Using part of the butter, grease large casserole dish. Melt the remaining butter and mix into the rice. Add all remaining ingredients and mix well. Bake at 325° Fahrenheit for 45 minutes or until lightly browned on top.

Makes about six servings

Training Food Recipes

Sports Drink Recipe
- 2 cups water
- 2 tsp sugar
- ⅛ tsp salt
- Splash of fruit juice

Mix all ingredients and shake well.

Homemade Energy Bars
- 3 cups rolled oats
- 1 cup granola (choose a variety without hydrogenated oils or high-fructose corn syrup)
- ½ cup sliced almonds
- ¼ cup peanut butter
- ¼ cup vegetable oil
- Two eggs
- 1 cup dried fruit (small bits, any variety)
- 1 cup honey
- ½ cup nonfat dry milk
- 2 tsp vanilla extract
- 1 tsp salt

For chocolate energy bars add ⅓ cup cocoa powder and reduce nonfat dry milk to ⅓ cup.

Heat oven to 350° Fahrenheit. Prepare a shallow oven tray or cookie sheet with waxed paper (spray the paper with cooking spray). Combine oats, granola, nuts, and dried fruit in a bowl. Mix in eggs and nonfat dry milk. Place vanilla, honey, oil, peanut butter, and salt in pan and simmer for 3 minutes. Combine all ingredients into the bowl and mix well. Press onto tray and bake for 30 to 35 minutes. Gently mark indentations for the bars and then allow them to harden for 30 minutes or longer.

Additional Nutrition Websites and Resources

Academy of Nutrition and Dietetics (formerly the American Dietetics Association ADA)

The Academy provides information for nutrition specialists as well as the public and provides additional links to credible nutrition resources and professionals in your area. Use the SCAN website can to find a sports dietitian close to you.
www.eatright.org
www.scandpg.org

American College of Sports Medicine (ACSM)

One of the foremost authorities on sports medicine and nutrition. The ACSM website provides a wealth of sports- and health-related information that can be accessed by the public.
http://acsm.org/access-public-information/acsm%27s-sports-performance-center
http://acsm.org/access-public-information/brochures-fact-sheets/fact-sheets

The Australian Institute of Sport

This website provides "Fact Sheets" for different supplements and a useful supplement classification system.
http://www.ausport.gov.au/ais/nutrition/supplements/classification

Fruits & Veggies More Matters

This website provides healthy recipes for kids and includes recipes that focus on fruits, vegetables, whole grains, and healthy protein sources. There are also great tips for getting children and adolescent involved in the kitchen!
http://www.fruitsandveggiesmorematters.org/kid-friendly-healthy-recipes

The National Collegiate Athletic Association (NCAA)

This website provides resources for nutrition and performance for collegiate athletes, and also includes information on banned substances for collegiate athletes.
http://www.ncaa.org/health-and-safety/nutrition-and-performance

The United States Anti-Doping Agency (USADA)

The agency's website provides the most up-to-date information on illegal and banned substances as well as a "Supplement 411" online tutorial.
http://www.usada.org/

United States Department of Agriculture (USDA)

The USDA's "choose my plate" website provides the latest nutrition recommendations and dietary guidelines. It also provides Internet-based activity and food trackers.
http://www.choosemyplate.gov

About the Author

Abigail J. Larson received her PhD in Exercise Science from the University of Utah and specializes in the physiology of exercise in athletes as well as clinical populations. Additionally, she has multiple degrees in nutrition and is a Registered Dietitian Nutritionist and Certified Specialist in Sport Dietetics. Originally from Minnesota, Abigail made her home in Cedar City, Utah after many years of education and sport-related wandering. Currently, as an Assistant Professor at Southern Utah University, Abigail teaches concepts and applications of exercise and clinical physiology as well as sport psychology and sport nutrition. Abigail has published numerous articles on the topics of sport conditioning and nutrition; her first text *Fuel for Sport* was published by Momentum Press in 2016. Abigail is also a former professional athlete and represented the US Ski Team as an Olympic athlete in Torino Italy (2006).

Kary Woodruff is a Certified Specialist in Sports Nutrition (CSSD) and Associate Instructor in the Department of Nutrition and Integrative Physiology at the University of Utah. She teaches Nutrition through the Lifecycle, Eating Disorders: Prevention and Treatment, and Women's Health and Nutrition. Kary also works as a sports dietitian at the LiVe Well Center in Salt Lake City and specializes in helping those with eating disorders. Kary is also on the United States Olympic Committee registry of sports dietitians and regularly works with elite athletes. Kary's education includes a Masters in Sports Psychology and a Masters in Sports Nutrition from the University of Utah, as well as a Bachelors in Psychology from the University of Massachusetts Amherst. Kary published the textbook 'Sports Nutrition' (publisher Momentum Press, 2016) and is a contributing author of Nutrition and Physical Fitness in the textbook 'Williams' Basic Nutrition & Diet Therapy' 15th edition.'

Index

Weight loss, in athletes
  diet, 57
  energy deficit, 58
  energy density, 58–59
  practices, 55–56
  weight management, 56–57
  weight measurements, 57
Weight-sensitive sports, 64
Whole grains, 5
World Anti-Doping Agency
    (WADA), 84

World Health Organization
    (WHO), 4

Yogurt-herb dip, 100

Zinc
  as antioxidants and immune system
    supporter, 28
  red blood cells production, 27

OTHER TITLES IN OUR HEALTH, WELLNESS, AND EXERCISE SCIENCE COLLECTION

Abigail J. Larson, *Editor*

- *Fuel for Sport: The Basics* by Abigail J. Larson
- *Strategies for Sport Nutrition Success: A Practical Guide to Improving Performance Through Nutrition* by Abigail J. Larson
- *Injury Recognition and Prevention: Lower and Upper Extremity* by Genevieve Ludwig and Megan Streveler

Momentum Press offers over 30 collections including Aerospace, Biomedical, Civil, Environmental, Nanomaterials, Geotechnical, and many others. We are a leading book publisher in the field of engineering, mathematics, health, and applied sciences.

Momentum Press is actively seeking collection editors as well as authors. For more information about becoming an MP author or collection editor, please visit http://www.momentumpress.net/contact

Announcing Digital Content Crafted by Librarians

Concise e-books business students need for classroom and research

Momentum Press offers digital content as authoritative treatments of advanced engineering topics by leaders in their field. Hosted on ebrary, MP provides practitioners, researchers, faculty, and students in engineering, science, and industry with innovative electronic content in sensors and controls engineering, advanced energy engineering, manufacturing, and materials science.

Momentum Press offers library-friendly terms:
- *perpetual access for a one-time fee*
- *no subscriptions or access fees required*
- *unlimited concurrent usage permitted*
- *downloadable PDFs provided*
- *free MARC records included*
- *free trials*

The **Momentum Press** digital library is very affordable, with no obligation to buy in future years.

For more information, please visit **www.momentumpress.net/library** or to set up a trial in the US, please contact **mpsales@globalepress.com**.

www.ingramcontent.com/pod-product-compliance
Lightning Source LLC
Chambersburg PA
CBHW050535270326

41926CB00015B/3239